W0050395

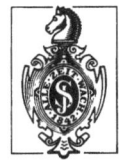

Werner Mendling

Vulvovaginal Candidosis

Theory and Practice

Foreword by H. Rieth

With 168 Figures, Most in Color

Springer-Verlag Berlin Heidelberg New York
London Paris Tokyo

Dr. Werner Mendling
Frauenklinik der Kliniken St. Antonius gGmbH
Vogelsangstraße 106
D-5600 Wuppertal 1

Translated by
Dora Wirth Languages Ltd
85 Campden Street
Kensington, London W8 7EN
England

Translation of "Die Vulvovaginalkandidose"
Kliniktaschenbücher, 1987
ISBN-13:978-3-540-18704-2

ISBN-13:978-3-540-18704-2   e-ISBN-13:978-3-642-83312-0
DOI: 10.1007/978-3-642-83312-0

This work is subject to copyright. All rights are reserved, whether the whole or part of the material is
concerned, specifically the rights of translation, reprinting, reuse of illustrations, recitation,
broadcasting, reproduction on microfilms or in other ways, and storage in data banks. Duplication of
this publication or parts thereof is only permitted under the provisions of the German Copyright Law
of September 9, 1965, in its version of June 24, 1985, and a copyright fee must always be paid.
Violations fall under the prosecution act of the German Copyright Law.
© Springer-Verlag Berlin Heidelberg 1988

The use of registered names, trademarks, etc. in this publication does not imply, even in the absence
of a specific statement, that such names are exempt from the relevant protective laws and regulations
and therefore free for general use.
Product Liability: The publisher can give no guarantee for information about drug dosage and
application thereof contained in the book. On every individual case the respective user must check its
accuracy by consulting other pharmaceutical literature.

2127/3145-543210

Foreword

The very rapid progress in gynaecological mycology in the last 15 years is of benefit not only to women with fungal infections but also to neonates who – to formulate it somewhat overdone – are "entitled to a fungus-free birth canal".

The development began 35 years ago at the Frauenklinik Finkenau, a Hamburg gynaecological hospital. The Director was Prof. Hanns Dietel. Collaboration with the Mycological Laboratory of the Universitäts-Hautklinik Hamburg-Eppendorf resulted in the formation of a germ cell of Gynaecological Mycology. Its products included Rüther, Behn, Malicke and Schnell.

Prof. Joseph Kimmig, a chemist and Professor of Dermatology, ushered in a new era with the synthesis of many benzimidazoles that proved highly potent against fungi pathogenic to man. His research formed the bedrock for the development of ever more effective antibiotics.

The therapeutic advances were paralleled by postgraduate and advanced training of gynaecologists in the field of genital mycoses. This is a task that Werner Mendling has made his own in a way that must reflect great credit on his teacher, Prof. Schnell.

The present paper will be of equal service to physicians in hospital or practice. It is absolutely up to date, concise and precise, stimulates thought and action and will help to ensure that in a case of mycosis, it is man, not the fungus, that comes out on top.

Hamburg-Eppendorf, January 1988
Professor Dr. med. Dr. med. vet. h. c. HANS RIETH

Preface

When, in 1976, I was a young intern at what was then the Rheinische Landesfrauenklinik und Hebammenlehranstalt Wuppertal – which despite a change in name and governance remains my gynaecological and obstetrical homeground – I curiously inspected some yeast cultures. The head physician, Dr. Schnell, thereupon suggested that I could do worse than take a real interest in this field. I took his advice, perhaps having a hunch that there were many ambitious colleagues who would find this rather too modest a subject. When I began to search for literature and practical information, I soon found that there was virtually nothing to help the beginner to get a quick grasp of the overall situation, the more so as mycology had been treated rather as a poor relation at my medical college.

And so, after the early departure of Dr. Schnell, I began to culture my own yeasts in a corner of the clinical laboratory. Although I engaged in this pursuit as constantly as was compatible with my fairly comprehensive clinical work, it went unnoticed by many of my colleagues.

I take this opportunity of thanking Prof. Dr. med. J. D. Schnell for introducing me to gynaecological mycology. At the same time, I find it rather sad than in the last ten years I never once met a colleague, male or female, who shared my interest in this fascinating and comprehensible subject.

Unless I wanted to give up this work, I simply had to build up my own experience.

I am particularly indebted to my two clinical teachers, Prof. Dr. med. H. Meinrenken and – for the last three years – Prof. Dr. med. H. Rüttgers, both of whom, each in his own way, kindly and generously permitted and encouraged "the spread of fungi" in their hospital.

In a large hospital, geared to practical work rather than research, such extra activities would – from organizational as well as the financial aspects – have hardly been feasible without assistance, the more so as I could only engage in them in my spare time.

I am therefore conscious of my good fortune and very grateful to the Head of the Mykologische Labor am Pharma-Forschungszentrum of Bayer AG, Dr. rer. nat. M. Plempel, and to his assistants, Frau B. Patschorke and Frau U. Lummerzheim, for their friendship and generosity at all times in helping me with materials, literature, knowledge, and with contacts.

It was almost inevitable that the increased medical interest in fungal diseases would prompt demands for postgraduate training, demands which have meanwhile been realized by about a hundred gynaecological-mycological seminars held in Germany and other countries. This in turn has given rise to the recurrent question by participants of where they could read up on what they had just seen or heard.

This little book is intended to meet these requirements and to fill the gap that faced me ten years ago. I have endeavored to convey the current – but rapidly increasing – state of knowledge in word and picture to the scientific and practical interest. Last but not least, the book is designed to meet the requirements of the general practitioners, which are not always adequately considered in postgraduate courses.

I shall be grateful for any comments on errors of omission or commission.

Wuppertal, March 1987
WERNER MENDLING

Table of Contents

1 General Outline

Fungi play a major part in medicine; their importance is growing and they are increasingly attracting the interest of the medical profession. Pulmonary **mycoallergies,** as for instance caused by molds or yeasts, are now more frequently recognised.

Mycotoxicoses are caused by toxic metabolic products of fungi (for instance, the hepatotoxic aflatoxin B_1 of *Aspergillus flavus*). According to press reports mycotoxins have even achieved military significance as agents in chemical warfare.

The term **mycetism** is applied to the ingestion of poisonous cap-forming fungi (basidiomycetes) either accidentally or deliberately (psychedelic fungi).

However, the "daily bread" of the gynecologist consists of the **mycoses,** which may be primary or secondary (candidosis as an "illness of the ill"). It is conceivable that every vaginal mycosis is a secondary mycosis even if the predisposing factor is not always apparent. Colonization of the intestine by large numbers of fungi may cause symptoms as a result of alcoholic fermentation without the presence of a mycosis in the strict sense of the word.

Modern medical mycology employs the classification of dermatophytes, yeasts and molds (and other fungi) (D-Y-M system based on Rieth 1967). Dermatophytes are almost never diagnosed as pathogens in the genital region although species of *Microsporum, Trichophyton rubrum* and *Trichophyton mentagrophytes* as well as *Epidermophyton floccosum* are rare causes of dermatophytoses of the vulva (Grimmer 1969). The diagnosis can only be made by culture and should be left to a physician experienced in mycology.

A rare case of trichophytosis of the mammary gland has been described after it was initially misdiagnosed as inflammatory breast carcinoma (Huhn and Stock 1977).

There are no confirmed reports of gynecological disorders caused by species of *Aspergillus* or *Penicillium*. Molds have in rare instances been demonstrated in vaginal secretions but without causing clinical illness (Schnell and Plempel 1972). The interpretation of direct wet mounts prepared with saline calls for care as mycelia and conidia of airborne *Penicillium* species may contaminate saline bottles for weeks or months and so become a permanent source of wrong diagnoses (Fig. 117).

Geotrichum candidum, a yeast-like mold that is a common, generally harmless inhabitant of the intestine, is very occasionally isolated from vaginal secretions, without discernible signs of illness.

Geotrichum candidum can be grown on Sabouraud's 2% glucose agar and forms white colonies with short aerial mycelia (see Fig. 80). Under the microscope, it is possible to distinguish mycelia – especially on rice agar – which may break up into short segments that look like budding cells (arthrospores) (see Fig. 81–83).

The so-called pseudomycoses (Meinhof 1977) – which are caused by microorganisms resembling fungi – include the important actinomycosis, which is most often caused by *Actinomyces israeli*. The organism may be present in the oral or the gastrointestinal flora. The typical sites of genital infections are the adnexa or parametrium where granulomatous lesions may develop. The condition is favored by intrauterine devices. The treatment, besides surgical intervention, includes high doses of penicillin for weeks or months (Ritzerfeld 1972).

Malassezia furfur is a dimorphic, imperfect fungus (deuteromycete) which of late is sometimes classified as a member of the *Cryptococcaceae* (Kreger-van Rij 1984). It occurs in a yeast stage and a mycelial stage and is the causative organism of pityriasis versicolor, which causes yellowish-brown scales and occasionally occurs in the genitocrural region.

Malassezia furfur cannot be cultured on the standard agars but requires a glucose-peptone-yeast extract agar overlaid with olive oil (Kreger-van Rij 1984).

Erythrasma is caused by *Corynbebacterium minutissimum* and is characterized by sharply marginated reddish-brown spots. The condition, like pityriasis versicolor, can be treated with imidazole derivatives.

Intertrigo, a dermatitis caused by friction and sweating (see Fig. 161), for instance in the groin, may obviously develop into a mycosis as a result of superinfection.

In general, however, gynecologists are faced with colonization and infection by facultative pathogenic opportunists, namely the imperfect yeasts, which be dealt with in detail below.

According to a recommendation by Yarrow and Meyer (1978) *Candida* and *Torulopsis* species should be combined in the genus *Candida* as *Torulopsis* spp. are occasionally capable of forming a (sparse) pseudomycelium (see Fig. 62). This idea was accepted, on application, by the Centraalbureau voor Schimmelcultures in Delft (L. Rodriguez de Miranda, personal communication 1985) and this classification is included in the new edition of the book previously edited by Lodder (Kreger-van Rij, 1984). However, there are currently still other suggestions concerning the allocation and classification of different yeasts (e.g. Barnett et al. 1986).

There are yeasts which under certain conditions can, by cell fusion, form several intracellular ascospores as fruiting bodies (ascosporogenic yeasts). These are accordingly classified as perfect yeasts: class *Ascomycetes,* order *Endomycetales* (yeasts in the wider sense), family *Saccharomycetaceae* (yeasts in the strict sense) (Preusser 1982). The family includes baker's yeast, *Saccharomyces cerevisiae* (see Figures 75-79). It is not normally regarded as pathogenic but there is some reason to question this on the basis of isolated references in the literature (Eng et al. 1984); furthermore, one of the author's own patients suffered from mild vaginal pruritus for several months. In the case of this patient, it was possible to demonstrate a clean lactobacillus flora of purity grade I according to Jirovec (1948). Yeasts were cultured on Sabouraud's 2% glucose agar. Topical treatment with clotrimazole eliminated neither the yeasts nor the symptoms which prompted species identification. *Saccharomyces cerevisae* was identified by culture, i. e. the formation of ascospores on rice agar, and the use of the API-20C Auxanogramme System. Further treatment for twelve days caused the yeast to disappear from the vagina and the patient was asymptomatic for the first time.

Saccharomyces cerevisae is occasionally cultured from the vaginal secretions of asymptomatic women. In a sample of our own patients, the organism was demonstrated in 0.7% of 283 pregnant women with yeast infections who were subjected to culture tests before entering the labour room and it also occurred in 0.9% of 214 non-pregnant women. Such accidental findings probably do not require treatment even if the species is identified – which is not normally the case under practice conditions.

No ascospore formation has so far been observed in other yeasts and they are accordingly classified as asporogenic, imperfect yeasts. The genera of the family *Cryptococcaceae* classified as imperfect yeasts include *Aciculoconidium, Brettanomyces, Candida, Cryptococcus, Kloeckera, Malassezia, Oosporidium, Phaffia, Rhodotorula, Sarcinosporum, Schizoblastosporium, Sterigmatomyces, Sympodiomyces, Trichosporon* and *Trigonopsis* (Kreger-van Rij 1984).

Candida species (including those formerly known as *Torulopsis*) and *Rhodotorula* spp. are those most commonly isolated from the vulvovaginal region. Rarely, *Trichosporon cutaneum (beigelii)* (s. Fig. 72–74) or *Geotrichum candidum,* a yeast-like mold are found (s. Fig. 80–83). *Candida* spp. are the only ones with any relevance as pathogens. At the present time, Kreger-van Rij (1984) describes 196 known species of Candida whereas Lodder, in 1971, listed only 81 species. However, according to Barnett et al. (1986) 155 yeast species should listed to the genus Candida.

Almost all *Candida* species are regarded as non-pathogenic and some are used in industry (Scientific American 11, 1981), e.g. *Candida kefyr, Candida utilis, Candida lipolytica* and others. Only 18 species of yeast have so far been recognised as facultative pathogens (Table 1); the eatable *Candida kefyr* is of late being regarded as identical with the facultatively pathogenic *Candida pseudotropicalis* (Kreger-van Rij 1984).

Yeasts, especially *Candida albicans,* can cause the disorders listed in Table 2.

The International Society for Human and Animal Mycology (ISHAM) and the Council for International Organization of Medical Sciences (CIOMS), both collaborating with the World Health

Table 1. Facultatively pathogenic imperfect yeasts (modified version of Rieth, 1979, 1984; Kreger-van Rij 1984)

Candida albicans (incl. *Candida stellatoidea*)	*Candida dattila* (formerly *Torulopsis dattila*)
Candida catenulata (formerly *Candida brumptii*)	*Candida famata* (formerly *Torulopsis candida*)
Candida guilliermondii	*Candida glabrata* (formerly *Torulopsis glabrata*)
Candida intermedia	
Candida kefyr (formerly *Candida pseudotropicalis*)	*Candida inconspicua* (formerly *Torulopsis inconspicua*)
Candida krusei	
Candida lusitaniae[a] (Terreni et al., 1986)	*Rhodotorula rubra*[a] *Cryptococcus neoformans*[a]
Candida parapsilosis	*Trichosporon cutaneum*[a]
Candida pulcherrima[a] (Weber and Kolb 1986; Begemann and Splanemann 1986)	
Candida tropicalis	
Candida zeylanoides	

[a] There is no evidence that these yeasts cause **vaginal mycoses.**

Table 2. Yeast infections that can be caused by *Candida* spp. in man (from Preusser 1982)

	Disorders of the Mucous Membranes	Skin Diseases	Systemic Diseases
Infections	Glossitis Stomatitis Cheilitis Perlèche Colpitis Balanitis Bronchitis Pneumonia Esophagitis Enteritis Periproctitis	Dermatitis Paronychia Onychomycosis Granuloma	Urogenital candidosis Endocarditis Meningitis Encephalitis Septicemia
Allergic conditions		Lesions caused by metabolites, eczema	Asthma Gastritis

Organization (WHO) independently published lists of names for the mycoses: the Nomenclature of Mycoses (1980) and International Nomenclature of Diseases (1982) (Löffler 1983) contain the correct term "candidose" in french and german language and illogically "candidiasis" in english.

2 The Incidence of Yeasts in Man

Yeasts of all types have a worldwide distribution. Their chief reservoirs are the skins and mucous membranes of man, mammals and birds and some also occur on fruits (Odds 1979).

Such facultatively opportunistic pathogens cannot be regarded as belonging to the normal body flora as, despite their frequent colonization of man, they by no means occur in every human subject. The colonization of man does not appear to have increased in recent decades (Odds 1979, Schnell 1982) but it does seem that changes in living conditions and certain aspects of modern medicine have caused certain high risk groups to become more predisposed to infection (infection = colonization plus disposition).

The principal predisposing factors include:

1. The increase in the regular consumption, beginning in infancy, of confectionary containing sugar and other carbohydrates which provide the fungi with nutrients in the intestine.
2. Increased medical intervention in some groups of patients, e.g. antibiotic therapy and the use of immunosuppressants in transplant surgery and oncology.
3. Greater longevity necessitating specialist care that allows yeasts to thrive on skin and mucous membranes.

The colonization of normal body skin by non-pathogenic or facultatively pathogenic yeasts increases with advancing age in healthy men and women. The incidence of *Candida albicans* is normally about 5% (Rieth 1979). Oehlschlägel et al. (1985), who examined a sample of 135 men and women, found that in 44.2% healthy skin was colonized by *Candida glabrata* or other species of *Torulopsis* (to use their former name) and other facultatively pathogenic species of *Candida* were demonstrated in 19.4%.

Candida albicans occurs in the oral cavity of every other healthy person (Odds 1979); this has been the case for decades throughout the world and even primitive societies are not exempt (Heber et al. 1975). People with dental prostheses or dental caries almost always harbor facultatively pathogenic yeasts (Spiechowicz and Weyman-Rzucidlo 1971, Vandenbussche and Swinne 1984). The presence of fungi, without any effect on the concomitant bacterial flora, causes a local reduction in the pH of the oral cavity and thus favors the development of carcinogenic N-nitroso compounds (Broschinski et al. 1986).

The gastrointestinal tract is known to be an important reservoir of yeasts (Vanbreuseghem 1970; Koch and Koch 1981; Fegeler et al. 1983), aided by the fact that the gastric hydrochloric acid seems to have hardly any adverse effects on *Candida albicans* (Meinhof 1974). The presence of facultatively pathogenic yeasts is demonstrated in, on average, 20–30% of all rectal examinations or fecal analyses (Benham and Hopkins 1933; Blaschke-Hellmessen et al. 1979, Odds 1979). Yeasts in the intestine may reach the bloodstream by "persorption" (Volkheimer 1967, Korte et al. 1968, Krause et al. 1969). Their presence in a blood culture, however, is not necessarily evidence of sepsis as a healthy body can eliminate a certain number of yeast cells without the aid of drugs. Conversely, in a case of yeast sepsis, it is often easier to demonstrate the pathogen in the urine than in the blood.

3 Genital Colonization in the Female Sex

Vaginal colonization by yeasts appear to be relatively rare in prepubertal children (Lang 1959, Heinz and Hoyme 1974, Huber 1977, Dewhurst 1980) although the feces of children may show the same contamination rates as those of adults (Di Menna 1954). Vulvovaginal mycoses are accordingly rare in children (see Fig. 147). It would seem that the low hormone levels, and thus the low sugar levels of the vagina in childhood offer conditions unfavorable for yeasts. However, when vulvovaginal mycosis is diagnosed in a child, it should prompt a thorough investigation for (immunosuppressant) disease or diabetes mellitus.

Yeasts are normally demonstrated in 5 to 10% of healthy postmenopausal women; this figure re-approximates the prepubertal levels

Table 3. Average incidence of facultatively pathogenic yeasts in the vagina

Patient Group	Incidence
Prepubertal children	"rarely" (3–5%)
Healthy non-pregnant premenopausal women	10%
Pregnant women	30%
Healthy postmenopausal women	5–10%
Non-pregnant women with weakening of the immune system caused by illness or due to the effects of hormones, drugs or other factors	min. 30%
226 women of an unselected autopsy material[a]	46%

[a] Study carried out at the Institut für Pathologie der Stadt Wuppertal (Rätz-Günther et al. 1987).

Table 4. Spectrum of yeast species isolated from the vaginas of different patient groups. To facilitate comparison, the figures represent the combined species counts from the original papers (expressed in %)

Authors	Kimmig and Rieth (1961)	Kimmig and Rieth (1961)	Schnell (1972)	Sonck (1978)	Jenny (1984)	Mendling (1984)	Mendling (1984)	Rätz-Günther et al. (1987)
Place	Hamburg	Hamburg	Wuppertal	Turku	Zurich	Wuppertal	Wuppertal and Duisburg	Wuppertal
Patient group	Women n	Vaginal mycoses	Cancer prophylaxis	Vaginal mycoses	Mixed	Vaginal mycoses	Women on day of parturition	Autopsy material
Isolated strains (n = 100%)	691	95	218	2003	242	81	283	93
Candida albicans	68.6	64.3	57.8	63.6	76.8	77.7	77.3	53.7
Other *Candida* spp.	11.7	9.4	17.4	6.5	2.3	6.1	11.9	15.0
Torulopsis glabrata and other *Torulopsis* spp.	13.0	14.8	24.8	9.0	12.7	14.7	7.7	30.1
Rhodotorula rubra, Saccharomyces cerevisae, Geotrichum candidum etc.	6.7	11.6				1.2	3.1	1.2

(Schnell et al. 1972, Mendling et al. 1979). The worldwide incidence of yeasts in the vaginas of healthy non-pregnant women of reproductive age is approximately 10% (Odds 1979, Schnell 1982) (Table 3).

The distribution of species of yeasts in the genital organs of healthy subjects is similar with negligible differences (Tables 4 and 5). *Candida albicans* has been shown to be the most commonly occurring yeast, with *Candida glabrata (Torulopsis glabrata)* in second place. The presence of typical risk factors (Table 6) results in a substantial increase in yeast colonization of the vagina. The incidence in non-pregnant women with gynecological disorders averages at least 30% (Schnell 1982). This is accompanied by an increase in the percentage of *Candida albicans* at the expense of other species, especially *Candida glabrata.*

We found in one of our own investigations that in a sample of 113 patients with carcinoma of the uterus, the incidence of yeast colonization of the vaginae was trebled from an initial 9.7% to 30.9% in the course of treatment with radium or radium-telecobalt (Mendling et al. 1979). This result is in accordance with the findings of other authors who in cytological (Meisels 1969) and cultural (Richter et al. 1977) studies initially found no increase in the incidence of yeasts in precancerous conditions of the cervix. In the case of invasive cervical carcinoma, the incidence of yeast colonizations actually decreased slightly as the disease progressed (probably due to less favourable local conditions). Intensive radiotherapy, however, caused a marked rise in the incidence of yeast invasions although the standard doses of radiation may inhibit the growth of yeasts (Mendling and Haller 1977). No association between yeasts and the development of cervical cancer has so far been established. Carcinogens have, however, been definitely demonstrated in *Candida parapsilosis,* which occasionally occurs in the vagina as a facultatively pathogenic yeast; the association of carcinogens with *Candida albicans* is regarded as probable (Blank et al. 1968; Rieth 1984).

An mycological-histological study initiated by the author on unselected autopsy material revealed colonizations of vagina, cervix uteri (!), urinary bladder and/or the colon by *Candida albicans, Candida glabrata* and some other yeasts in 20 to 50% of cases. In

Table 5. Spectrum of yeast species isolated from the vaginas in a mixed sample of many women with and in a few cases without vaginal mycoses (Frauenklinik Wuppertal 1986)

Isolated strains	n 214	% 100
a) Facultatively pathogenic yeasts[a]		
Candida albicans	169	78.9
Candida glabrata	19	8.8
Candida quilliermondii or famata[b]	8	3.7
Candida krusei	4	1.8
Candida species	4	1.8
Candida tropicalis	2	0.9
Candida famata	2	0.9
Candida parapsilosis	1	0.4
b) Non-pathogenic yeasts[a]		
Candida lusitaniae	1	0.4
Rhodotorula rubra	1	0.4
Trichosporon capitatum	1	0.4
Saccharomyces cerevisiae	2	0.9

[a] concerning vaginal infections.
[b] These yeasts cannot always be reliably differentiated on rice agar or with the API 20C Auxanogramme System.

Table 6. Factors that can predispose to yeast infection

Exogenous	Endogenous
Oral contraceptives high in gestagens	Metabolic disorders e.g.
Treatment with	Diabetes mellitus
– gestagens, antiandrogens, corticosteroids;	Cushing's disease
– immunosuppressants or cytotoxic drugs	Addison's disease
– broad-spectrum antibiotics;	Hypothyroidism, hyperthyroidism
– metronidazole?	Iron deficiency?
Radiotherapy	Debilitating diseases that weaken the immune system, e.g. leukemia,
Yeast harbored by sexual partner	acquired immune deficiency syndrome
Orogenital or anogenital intercourse	(AIDS) etc.
Occupation (work at swimming pools, innkeeper, hospital nurse etc.)	
Diet rich in carbohydrates	

autopsies on men the same yeasts, with similar incidences, were recovered from the penis, prostate, seminal vesicles and/or the urinary bladder, generally without any signs of a mycosis except one case of urethrocystitis in a woman and one case of prostatitis! (Rätz-Günther et al. 1987).

Diabetics are known to be particularly susceptible to candidoses [as well as torulopsidoses (Wegmann 1979)]. Glucose stimulates the formation of budding cells of *Candida albicans* and insulin, even at normal glucose levels, activates the formation of germ tubes and pseudomycelia and thus aids the transition from colonization to infection (Nolting et al. 1982). Different views have been published on cell-mediated immunity and phagocytosis of *Candida albicans* in diabetics (Odds 1979). Raith et al. (1983) came to the conclusion that the granulocytes of diabetics were less effective than those of healthy subjects in killing *Candida albicans*.

Corticosteroids, immunosuppressants and cytotoxic agents reduce the natural defences of the body and their prolonged use predisposes to all kinds of infection. The effects of various standard cytotoxic agents on *Candida albicans* have been investigated *in vitro* (Ghannoum and Al-Khars 1984). Inhibitory activities, lysis and an increased incidence of atypical pseudomycelia were observed in most cases. It may thus be assumed that in view of the apparently detrimental effects of these drugs on yeasts, the latters' increased incidence during treatment with cytotoxic agents must be attributable solely to the lowered resistance of the patients.

A newly recognised disease, the acquired immune deficiency syndrome (AIDS), is associated with a disposition for recurrent candidoses (Cran et al. 1985). A refractory candidosis of the tongue, in particular, should prompt screening for human immunodeficiency virus (HIV) (Klein et al. 1984).

Antibiotics are also thought to favour "levuroses" i. e. yeast infections; they appear to inhibit the synthesis of antibodies as well as phagocytic activity and thus to lower resistance to yeasts (Carlson and Husmann 1956, Seelig 1966). Clinical impressions have been confirmed by numerous reports and penicillins and tetracyclines in particular (Dukes and Tettenbaum 1954) are believed to stimulate fungal growth (Odds 1979). Heber et al. (1975), on the other hand, found no differences in the incidence of oral or genital yeast colonisation between soldiers treated with antibiotics and those not treated with antibiotics. McKenrick (quoted by Odds 1979) likewise, in the only known double-blind study comparing tetracyclines with placebo in 96 men with chronic bronchitis, found no significant difference in oral yeast colonization before and after treatment. The most recent *in-vitro* studies and animal experiments have shown that of various antibiotics tested, only tetracyclines caused a faster detachment of young budding cells from older groups of blastoconidia, resulting in an increase in the number of cells – but not the biomass – of *Candida albicans*. Animal studies also showed that broad-spectrum antibiotics did not result in dissemination of experimentally induced intestinal mycoses (Plempel 1986). It is conceivable, however, that the supposed antibiotic side-effects occur in a "selected" group of patients weakened as a result of infection in whom the antibiotic-induced elimination of the physiological flora allows the yeasts to adhere and cause infection "without hindrance". Conversely, some bacteria of the physiological flora, e.g. species of *Escherichia coli,* are capable of blocking the penetration of *Candida albicans* into the tissues.

Metronidazole, initially marketed as an antitrichomonal agent and now undergoing a revival as an anaerobicide, has been repeatedly reported to favour vaginal colonization by yeasts (Odds 1979). Bearing in mind the uses of metronidazole in gynecology, this phenomenon is difficult to interpret. Yeasts are isolated from approx. 10% of women with trichomoniasis (Schnell et al. 1972; Szarmach et al. 1983). Inspite of concomitant yeast colonization, concomitant yeast infection signs are rare in bacterial vaginosis (Czango 1982) or "aminocolpitis" (Petersen 1985). Trichomoniasis and bacterial vaginosis are similar in respect of both the predisposing factors and the effects on conditions in the vagina which are if anything detrimental to yeasts. There have, however, been incidents where treatment with metronidazole restored the lactobacilli but the patient complained of vaginal candidosis. It has still to be elucidated whether this is caused by metronidazole or rather by competition between bacteria and yeasts on the epithelial surfaces and lowering of resistance in the vagina which manifests itself by the presence of large numbers of bacteria and/or trichomonads and which, after elimination of these microorganisms, allows an existing, though small

14

number of yeast cells to proliferate. This concept of the author was supported by Monif (1985) by means of quantitative yeast-cell and bacterial counts in a patient who after bacterial vaginitis and its treatment with metronidazole exhibited a sharp rise in the vaginal yeast count followed by candidosis.

The administration of gestagens (Patt et al. 1972, Birnbaum and Kraussold 1975, Patt and Korte 1975) or antiandrogens (Farkas and Simon 1980) favours colonization by yeasts as do Cushing's disease and obesity. There have also been reports of an increased incidence of mycoses in patients with hyperthyroidism or hypothyroidism.

Particular attention should be paid to hormonal contraception. It is described in the literature as a typical risk factor for vaginal colonization by yeasts (Patt et al. 1972). Different estrogens and gestagens have been shown *in vitro* to have no stimulant effects on the growth of *Candida albicans* or *Candida glabrata* (Neumann and Kaben 1971, Schnell 1982), nor does the pH have a direct effect on fungal growth (Odds 1979; Schnell 1982). The view of most authors is that gestagens are the decisive factor in the proliferation of intravaginal yeasts. The increases in the shedding of cells and glycogen cleavage by lactobacilli mean that more glucose is made available to the yeasts. This effect, however, is no longer likely to have any real relevance as the newer preparations with low hormone contents are now generally prescribed. This impression was confirmed by Göttlicher and Madjaric (1983), who demonstrated a reducing trend in the incidence of yeast colonization of the vagina despite the use of oral contraceptives; the incidence was the same, approximately 17%, as in 1981 in a sample of 1004 of their patients who were not taking oral contraceptives.

Unfortunately these two authors based their findings only on direct preparations without the use of cultures but as the error rate is likely to have been the same in both samples and in view of the large number of cases, the two groups are readily comparable.

Cultures were used by Davidson and Oates (1985) who in London between 1976 and 1984 examined 1363 women using different contraceptives. They found the incidence of yeasts to be no higher in women taking oral contraceptives (Table 7).

There is some controversy as to whether the incidence of yeasts is higher in women with intra-uterine devices than in other healthy

Table 7. Incidence of vaginal colonization by yeasts in unselected women using different contraceptives (From Davidson and Oates)

	Women examined n	Yeasts isolated from vagina	
		n	%
Oral contraceptives	651	179	27.5
Intra-uterine device	145	37	25.5
Others (condoms, diaphragms, spermicides)	184	64	34.8
No contraception	383	106	27.7
Total	1363	386	28.3

women, in so far as any valid statement can be made at all on the basis of few studies and the lack of large samples or suitable culture methods (Birnbaum and Kraussold 1975; Knippenberger et al. 1979; Davidson and Oates 1985). In the cases of mycoses, however, women with intra-uterine devices are at a disadvantage, presumably because budding cells on the thread of the device can surmount the barrier of the cervical mucus and thus become a source of reinfection.

Vaginal tampons, if used correctly, do not normally affect the vaginal environment (Loch and Esser-Mittag 1985) but it was shown experimentally that proteolysis products of *Candida albicans* activated the growth of *Staphylococcus aureus*, *Escherichia coli* and various other microorganisms occurring in the vagina (Staib and Geier 1971). This could be of relevance in connection with the toxic shock syndrome occasionally described after the use of tampons.

Man-made fabrics and tight clothing may be regarded as favouring the growth of yeasts in the genital region (Bull 1969; Hurley 1975). Although the author knows of no scientific study to validate this observation, it seems plausible in view of the results of an investigation which showed the incidence of fungal colonization of the feet to be lower in wearers of sandals allowing free access of air (Nickerson et al. 1945).

Although the incidence of vaginal yeast colonisation is approximately the same in the warm and cold regions of the world, some authors, including Göttlicher and Madjaric (1983) have shown that in a substantial sample, yeasts were present significantly more often in the warm season. This was attributed to warmth, visits to swimming baths and more frequent sexual intercourse.

Most authors confirm the general risk of picking up fungi in swimming baths and saunas as mats and wooden grates tend to harbor dermatophytes, yeasts and molds, which emphasizes the need for effective means of disinfection. Although bathing suits and trunks that do not withstand boiling may conceivably be sources of reinfection for genital mycoses in susceptible subjects, most authors take the view that the relatively rare demonstration of *Candida albicans* in german swimming pools [Effendy and Schirrmeister (1985) quoted 3.1%, generally in changing rooms and women's lavatories] means that these sources have no major epidemiological importance.

Nevertheless, those working in bathing establishments as well as innkeepers, hospital nurses and housewives, are always being listed as running special occupational risks.

No precise investigations have been carried out on the incidence of nosocomial yeast infections in hospital patients. Daschner (1984), working on records from the United Kingdom, the United States and the Federal Republic of Germany, quoted *Candida albicans* as accounting for 3.2–4.7% of all hospital infections.

The cervix is probably an effective barrier against ascending yeasts (Lachenicht et al. 1976; Meinhof 1976); this seems to be borne out by the fact that no yeasts have so far been demonstrated as causes of ascending infections in the non-pregnant uterus or tubes. On the other hand, Rodriguez et al. (1972) reported a case history of candida endometritis. The diagnosis was made at hysterectomy after years of gestagen treatment and was based solely on the histological demonstration of mycelia so that a mycosis due to other causes cannot be definitely ruled out.

In cases of colonization of neonates, yeasts have been found on the nipples (Schnell 1982) and in breast milk (Kintzel et al. 1971) whilst they occurred only rarely in the mammary secretions of non-pregnant women (Wunderlich 1979). Candidosis of the nipples is exceedingly rare (Opri 1982) and consequently may give rise to initial misdiagnosis. Huhn and Stock (1977) – as mentioned above – described a case of granulomatous trichophytosis of the mammary gland which was initially diagnosed as breast cancer.

4 Yeasts in Pregnancy and Neonatal Mycoses

Colonization of the vagina by yeasts increases continuously from the beginning of pregnancy up to the date of parturition by which time yeasts are recovered from approx. 30% of all untreated women. If we accept the evidence of methodologically comparable case studies, based on adequate samples, from the current century (Patt et al. 1972; Odds 1979; Schnell 1982), it appears that this percentage has not changed since time immemorial. The pregnancy-induced changes appear to favor in particular *Candida albicans,* as the incidence of *Candida glabrata* is in fact lower than in non-pregnant healthy women (see Table 4).

Despite the higher incidence of yeasts in the vaginas of pregnant women they are, according to our experience, not much more likely to develop vaginal mycoses than non-pregnant women. Other authors hold different views, maintaining that the signs and symptoms of vaginitis are frequently present but are often misinterpreted due to pregnancy related effects such discharge, lividity and nonspecific pruritus (Carroll and Hurley 1973). Preclampsia, parity, age and nationality are not additional risk factors (Schnell 1982).

Although the lochia appear to stimulate the growth of *Candida albicans* and *Candida glabrata* in vitro (Neumann and Kaben 1972), vaginal yeast colonization tends to subside postpartum even without treatment (Schnell 1982). This observation was recorded as early as 1870 by Haussmann in Berlin, who was one of the first to publish a detailed description of vaginal colonization by yeasts and other pathogens, their infectivity and transmission to the neonate resulting in candidosis or "thrush." He also, as long ago as 1870, advocated prophylactic treatment of the vagina!

More recently, precise studies, based on cultures, have confirmed that yeasts harbored by the mother are transmitted to the child (Epstein 1924) and there are descriptions of the route of infection from the maternal vagina to the neonate in the course of vaginal delivery (Woodruff and Hesseltine 1938; Blaschke-Hellmessen 1968; Schnell 1975; Holtorff et al. 1976; Schwarze et al. 1976). Since that time at least, every neonate has been regarded as being "entitled to a fungus-free birth canal" (Rieth 1969).

Candida albicans is virtually an obligate pathogen for a healthy child in the first few days or weeks of life; colonization by yeasts before the end of the first week of life results in mycosis within 1 to 3 weeks in at least 90% of cases (Schnell 1982) with an almost equal incidence of oral candidosis (thrush, mycotic stomatitis) and anogenital candidosis (diaper dermatitis, napkin-area dermatitis) (Fig. 144–146).

According to Seebacher (1981) napkin-area dermatitis, infantile seborrhoic dermatitis and its most serious variant, erythrodermia desquamativa (Leiner's disease) represent the same disease caused by a yeast infection. This is often accompanied by a seborrhoic id-reaction, for instance, on the scalp of the child (candidid).

Blaschke-Hellmessen (1972) found that from the third week to the third year of life, only 9.7% of children harboring yeasts were asymptomatic. As the incidence of infection reaches its peak between 2 and 4 weeks, the children tend not to show any clinical signs in the first few days while they are still in hospital (Table 8). Extra vigilance on behalf of the hospital pediatrician or nurses and the resultant early diagnosis of neonatal fungal infection may, unfortunately, give rise in lay circles to the mistaken impression that fungal infections are exceptionally prevalent in the hospital concerned.

Fungal contamination of the mother's nipple – causing no symptoms – may be a source of reinfection for the child. In one case, described as a rarity, a lactating woman developed cutaneous candidosis of the nipple resulting from oral candidosis of the child (Nanjappa Chetty et al. 1980).

Preterm neonates receiving intensive care in an incubator are especially at risk and may die of candidal sepsis. The signs of the latter are nonspecific and the diagnosis, based on blood and urine cultures, cannot always be made in time. A deep mycosis caused by

Table 8. Incidence (based on the literature) of neonatal yeast infections (in percent) depending on the age of the child

Author	Year	Age of the Child (Days)							
		1	6	10	14	28	49	70	365
Valleix (quoted by Epstein 1924)	1839					25			
Fischl (quoted by Epstein 1924)	1883	1.75–2.5							
Epstein	1924	2.4					24.6		1
Plass, Hesseltine and Borts	1931			16.6					
Ludlam and Henderson (quoted by Schnell 1982)	1942			7.2					
Schwarze, Blaschke-Hellmessen, Hinkel, Hoffmann and Weigl	1976	3.0		11.5			13.0	9.5	4.5
Schnell	1982	1.4			6.1	10.7			

Candida albicans was established as the cause of death in 15 (1.8%) of 792 autopsies on neonates (Ziegler and Veith 1967). The diagnosis of fungal sepsis is still too often made by the pathologist (Brandt 1984).

There are very rare reports of intrauterine candidosis of a fetus with chorioamnionitis despite an intact amnion. Schnell (1982) found 34 cases in the literature since 1958 and added one case of his own. Grauwerky et al. (1983) published one further case but this involved premature rupture of the amnion. The route of infection is assumed to be through the cervix via the pole of the amnion despite the fact that amniotic fluid appears to inhibit the growth of *Candida albicans* (Jankowski et al. 1977). It is conceivable that there are exceptionally virulent strains that overcome such defenses. The inhibition of yeast growth by amniotic fluid was, however, also observed by Neumann and Kaben (1972).

In order to prevent neonatal mycoses, gynecologists should carry out vaginal examinations in good time (approx. 2–6 weeks before the estimated date of delivery). If the microscopic examination is negative, it should be followed by culture. If yeasts are detected, topical antifungal treatment has to be initiated. In connection with a study carried out by the author (Mendling and Schnell 1984), over half of 48 Wuppertal gynecologists stated that they carried out routine screening for fungi in pregnancy, including cultures. Of 456 German women questioned on the day of delivery, 9.6% stated that they had recently been treated for yeasts. Consequently yeasts were recovered from the vaginas of only 17.7%. Of 229 non-German, mostly Turkish, women, only 5.2% reported vaginal treatment with antifungal agents. Fungi were found in 28.8% of this group.

The incidence of antepartal vaginal yeast colonizations is normally the same in untreated women in Germany and other countries and this accordingly includes migrant workers in the Federal Republic of Germany (Odds 1979, Schnell 1982). It must be assumed that the reason for the higher incidence in the 229 – mostly Turkish – women investigated by us was due to problems of communication with their gynecologists and that furthermore, their religious and ethnic background made them reluctant to undergo genital examination in the course of treatment (Tatra 1973).

In the meantime Schnell (1986), by improved measures to eliminate yeasts from the vagina antepartum, reduced the incidence of yeasts at the time of parturition to 12% (54 of 448); *Candida albicans* was isolated from 7.1%.

It is accepted that the topical antifungal agents in current use, i.e. polyene or imidazole derivatives, have no adverse effects on the fetus. The use of these agents in treating the mother reduced the incidence of infantile infections to a minimum (Schnell 1982). Alternatively, the child has to be treated after the occurrence of symptoms and the demonstration of yeasts, which is less reliable. A routine prophylactic program for all neonates is not recommended.

5 Yeasts – Modes of Infection – Host Reactions

5.1 Candida albicans

Candida albicans (Robin) Berkhout (Fig. 3–10) described by Robin as *Oidium albicans* in 1853 and by Berkhout as *Candida albicans* in 1923, has had at least a hundred names bestowed on it down the years (Kreger-van Rij 1984). It is a dimorphic asporogenic yeast. *Candida albicans* can develop typical growth patterns in different *in vitro* and *in vivo* conditions as shown by Preusser (1982) in superb photographs. On peptone-glucose agar (e.g. Sabouraud's 2% glucose agar) *Candida albicans* normally grows in the form of round to oval budding cells (blastospores, Y = yeast form), approx. 4–8–10 μm in size (Fig. 5). Blastospores are regarded as saprophytic variants in the body. Macroscopically, colonies on Sabouraud's 2% glucose agar appear ivory in color, usually with a waxy sheen and without aerial mycelium. They have a typical odor.

So far, two different serotypes (A and B) have been clearly distinguished in morphologically and biochemically identical species of *Candida albicans*. Serotype A is the most widely distributed (Hasenclever and Mitchell 1961; Müller and Kirchhoff 1969). The serotypes appear to differ in their sensitivity to antifungal agents (Anger et al. 1984).

When *Candida albicans* is grown on rice agar low in nutrients by the method of Taschdjian (1953) and Rieth (1958) (Fig. 102) or on certain synthetic media (e.g. Meinhof 1975) and with reduced partial pressure of oxygen. (Preusser and Rostek 1983), under a cover slip at room temperature, it forms pseudomycelia (M = mycelial form) and large chlamydospores (double-walled resting spores)

(Fig. 7 and 8). These may be likened to a fingerprint as diagnostic criteria in the identification of these yeasts.

Candida stellatoidea (Fig. 11-14), a rare variant, is also able to form chlamydospores. It can be distinguished from *C. albicans* under the microscope by its protochlamydospores (Fig. 13 and 14). DNA investigations have meanwhile shown that *Candida albicans* and *Candida stellatoidea* are identical so that the latter should probably be regarded as no more than a morphological variant (from Meyer 1979, quoted in Kreger-van Rij 1984).

Pseudohyphae (Fig. 6-8, 110-114) are budding cells elongated by apical growth which, if they do not break up, can be distinguished by the "constrictions" between the cells. They are regarded as the infectious stage of the yeast in the body. *Candida albicans* occasionally forms a true "rope-ladder" mycelium which can be recognised under an electron microscope by its septa and the pores in the latter (Scherwitz et al. 1978).

The demonstration of yeast pseudohyphae or hyphae in host material is regarded as histological evidence of the presence of a mycosis.

Candida albicans forms germ tubes (Fig. 9 and 10) in serum and on certain agar media (Müller 1980). They are produced after only 1-4 hours as protrusions from budding cells without septa and may develop into mycelia (Taschdjian et al. 1960; Scherwitz and Rassner 1978).

The unequivocal differentiation of a particular yeast generally requires, besides identification of its morphological characteristics, an investigation of its sugar assimilation and sugar fermentation. *Candida albicans* induces fermentation of, for instance, glucose and maltose and assimilates these and other carbohydrates. These activities can be demonstrated by a number of commercially available kits, e.g. API 20 C Auxanogramme, Mérieux (Fig. 103 and 104); Uni Yeast-Tek plate, Flow Laboratories, and Mykotube Roche, Hoffmann-La Roche (Fig. 105).

The transition from colonization by a yeast to its actually causing disease involves in the first instance the adherence of budding cells to the superficial epithelial tissues (Kimura and Pearsall 1980; Sobel et al. 1981; Anderson and Odds 1985); the formation of germ tubes appears to have a significant role in this. *Candida albicans* has a stronger adhesive potential than other *Candida* spp. (King et al. 1980).

The formation of germ tubes can be stimulated *in vitro* by glucose or a pH of approx. 6, and inhibited by lactobacilli by way of a "coating effect". Studies using electron microscopy have illustrated the wormlike penetration of germ tubes into the host cells with unidentified matter being deposited at the site of contact (Farrell et al. 1983). Yeasts remaining in the budding-cell stage, on the other hand, never penetrated the walls of host cells and could be easily washed off. It appeared that the tip of a germ tube or a pseudohypha, like the point of a drill, was in some way especially equipped to pierce the wall of the host cell, possibly by the formation of a proteinase (Farrell, personal communication 1985). What conditions ultimately induce an existing yeast flora to cause an infection and thus disease have not yet been elucidated.

In the case of infections with *Candida albicans,* the budding cells and short pseudomycelia may penetrate the vaginal epithelium to a depth of 8–10 layers of cells with both intracellular and extracellular occurrence of yeast cells (Schnell and Voigt 1974). According to Rüther et al. (1958) and the author's own experience, histological studies using light microscopy in culturally confirmed vaginal mycoses tend to be unsatisfactory as only the most superficial epithelial layers are affected (Fig. 120, 121, 123) and in addition special staining methods are needed (e.g. Grocott's stain) to visualize the fungal elements (Fig. 122 and 124).

Vaginal candidoses obviously induce a local humoral response which manifests itself in raised antibody titers measurable in the vaginal and sometimes the cervical secretions and to a lesser extent also in the serum. Apart from IgG, IgA is the immunoglobulin most frequently found and because of its high titer locally, it is described as "secretory" IgA (Waldmann et al. 1971; Mathur et al. 1977; Syverson et al. 1979; Somos et al. 1982). Recently, Rakosi et al. (1986) also found a candida-specific IgE on the surface of yeast cells in patients with vaginal candidoses, which raises the possibility that an allergic phenomenon (pruritus!) may be involved.

However, it seems that the dominant part in cell-mediated defense against *Candida albicans* is played by the T-lymphocytes (Fegeler et al. 1978). Animal studies, on partially immune mice, showed marked host cell reactions by "activated" lymphocytes, macrophages and mast cells (Kuttin et al. 1984). Neutrophilic granulocytes can attack and destroy pseudomycelia (Diamond et al. 1978). *Candida* species with marked protease activity, such as *Candida albicans, Candida tropicalis* and *Candida parapsilosis* are more easily recognised and phagocytosed by polymorphonuclear neutrophils than those with weaker protease formation (Hauck et al. 1985; Walther et al. 1986). Protease activity is in turn dependent on an adequate supply of glucose and conversely can be inhibited *in vitro* by pepstatin (Schönborn 1984).

It appears that the phosphatase activity of some *Candida* species can also increase their pathogenicity (Farid et al. 1980).

The *in-vitro* results of Piccolella et al. (1981) are of particular interest. These suggest that the cell wall polysaccharides of *Candida albicans* through immunomodulation in the host can themselves affect pathogenicity by stimulating the maturation of T-suppressor lymphocytes.

In chronic vaginal candidosis, antigen-antibody complexes (asteroid bodies) can be demonstrated by electron microscopy on the outer cell wall of the fungi (Melchinger et al. 1980). Some studies stress the special importance of the complement and of the alternative pathway (properdin) in infections with *Candida albicans* or *Candida glabrata* (Grob and Wüthrich 1974; Ferrante and Thong 1979).

No increased incidence of candidosis was found in over 1000 patients with B-lymphocyte defects, including 80 patients lacking sIgA (Hobbs et al. 1977).

It would seem that the serum of healthy subjects contains a "*Candida albicans* killing factor" (Heite et al. 1964; Louria and Brayton 1964; Tomšíková and Novačková 1981) which is related to transferrin but not to humoral antibodies and which seems to be considerably reduced in diabetics.

5.2 Candida glabrata (Torulopsis glabrata)

Candida glabrata (Anderson) Meyer and Yarrow (formerly *Torulopsis glabrata*) is after *Candida albicans* the yeast most commonly isolated in vaginal mycoses (Fig. 57-62).

The yeast was described by Berlese in 1895 and referred to by Anderson in 1917 as *Cryptococcus glabratus;* Lodder and De Vries used the term *Torulopsis glabrata* in 1938 (Lodder 1971). Reference was made previously to the present-day inclusion of this yeast in the genus *Candida* by Yarrow and Meyer (1978) as well as by Kreger-Van Rij (1984).

Candida glabrata grows on Sabouraud's 2% glucose agar as whitish shiny colonies. The budding cells are mostly oval and, at approx. 3×5 μm, are markedly smaller than those of *Candida albicans*. Under a light microscope they often appear to have dark "pigmentation" and on rice agar they only occasionally form rudimentary pseudohyphae approx. 2-4 budding cells in length (Fig. 62).

No pseudomycelia were ever recovered from one of our own patients who has had recurrent mild symptoms from a vaginal infection with *Candida glabrata* for four years.

How *Candida glabrata* manages to cause symptoms and disease without forming pseudohyphae is not clear and investigations into the phenomenon are few or non-existent. These gaps in our knowledge cause special therapeutic problems.

6 Clinical Signs and Symptoms of Candida Vulvovaginitis

The clinical signs and symptoms of vulvovaginal mycoses are not always typical and occasionally deceptive. The most common pathogen is *Candida albicans* which accounts for approx. 75–80% of cases. Acute candidosis usually begins with itching which then turns to burning. A white to yellowish crumbly discharge (Fig. 125 and 127) is often but – especially in the early stages – not always present. There is typically a premenstrual worsening of the symptoms with alleviation after the menses. Dysuria and dyspareunia are inevitable consequences. The yeasts themselves do not change the pH. The vaginal flora of lactobacilli was found to be increased (!) in (all?) vaginal mycoses (Müller et al. 1981). In cases of acute vaginal candidosis, caused by *Candida albicans,* gynecological examination generally reveals florid or patchy redness of the vaginal wall and cervix (Fig. 128 and 129) and occasionally punctiform or patchy whitish exudates (Fig. 128) which if wiped off may leave erosions or bleeding areas. The symptoms cannot always be easily recognised in pregnancy since there is, in any case, an increase in the discharge and lividity. Mild pruritus and discharge are often reported in pregnancy without cultural demonstration of fungi (in one of our own studies, this applied to approximately one third of almost 700 patients in the third trimester).

The symptoms of vaginal mycosis may largely or completely subside even without treatment or cause considerable discomport for months; this is borne out by case histories (Mayer 1862; Winckel 1866; Haussmann 1870; Plass et al. 1931) and can occasionally be observed even today.

Vulvitis (Fig. 127–130) usually presents with marked redness and edema of the vulva which is tender and painful. The perianal region is often infected and reddened which is a sign of intestinal colonization (Fig. 132). An interesting phenomenon that has hardly been investigated so far is that some women always develop primary vulvitis without colpitis whilst in others, colpitis occurs without vulvitis although yeasts are isolated from both sites. This warrants a closer investigation of vulvitis and vaginitis from a dermatological viewpoint. Meech et al. (1985) succeeded in showing that in cases of hypersensitivity to intradermally administered cytoplasmic *Candida* antigens, even small numbers of yeast often cause vulvitis, especially after microtrauma (Table 9). Similar factors may apply to the corresponding condition in males (balanitis).

According to Monif (1985) diabetics are especially prone to candi-

Table 9. Clinical, microbiological and immunological findings in recurrent genital candidoses (modified from Meech 1985)

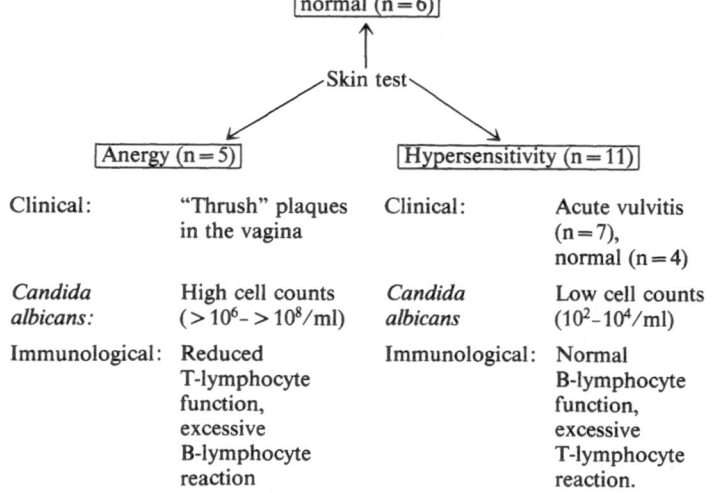

Clinical:	Yeasts and bacterial vaginosis
Candida albicans:	Varying cell counts (10^2 to $< 10^5$/ml)
Immunological:	Normal T- and B-lymphohocyte function

normal (n = 6)

Skin test

Anergy (n = 5)		Hypersensitivity (n = 11)	
Clinical:	"Thrush" plaques in the vagina	Clinical:	Acute vulvitis (n = 7), normal (n = 4)
Candida albicans:	High cell counts ($> 10^6$- $> 10^8$/ml)	*Candida albicans*	Low cell counts (10^2-10^4/ml)
Immunological:	Reduced T-lymphocyte function, excessive B-lymphocyte reaction	Immunological:	Normal B-lymphocyte function, excessive T-lymphocyte reaction.

dal vulvitis whereas candidal vaginitis occurs after antibiotic therapy. Grimmer (1968) distinguishes four forms of vulvomycosis:

- A vesicular form with discrete, later confluent yellowish vesicles surrounded by narrow erythematous margins (Fig. 130 and 131),
- An eczematous form (Fig. 136 and 137) with edema and red lesions with scaly margins and raised centres (in the author's view, this is a later stage – by a few days – of the vesicular form when the vesicles have been opened by scratching and friction),
- A follicular form with pustules and papules in the pubic hair follicles (Fig. 127),
- The extremely rare granulomatous form which begins as a chronic intracutaneous mycosis in childhood and which, as a consequence of granulomatous inflammatation, may give rise to verruciform hyperkeratotic nodules. It is associated with a defect in cell-mediated immunity which differs between individuals.

Vulvovaginal mycoses are occasionally associated with severe redness and pain in the ducts of Bartholin's glands which can obviously be involved. Fungi can also invade and infect the urethra and urinary bladder. Fungal cystitis is, however, rare (Hildick-Smith et al. 1964; Seneca 1968; Rieth 1970; Lipsky 1974). Yeasts isolated from mid-stream and even catheter urine in vulvovaginal mycoses generally emanate from the lower urethra or the vulva (Lachenicht and Potel 1976). Urine for the demonstration of yeasts should preferably be obtained by supra-pubic aspiration or possibly with the aid of a catheter: Lenzer (1978) recommends collection by cystoscopy with the aid of a loop developed by him. The findings are pathognomonic only if there are not less than 10,000 to 15,000 fungal cells per ml urine (Wise et al. 1976; Kozinn et al. 1978).

Urine acts as a nutrient medium for yeasts and must be examined at once (Owuso et al. 1978).

Wegman (1979) stressed that *Candida glabrata* also occurred more often in the urinary tracts of diabetics than of healthy subjects and that in concentrations exceeding 10^5/ml, it could cause cystitis or pyelonephritis.

The clinical signs and symptoms of vulvovaginal candidosis caused by *Candida albicans* or other *Candida* spp. tend to be similar. In view of the relative rarity of the involvement of, for instance, *Candida krusei* in vaginal mycosis, sufficient knowledge is not yet available concerning the clinical aspects, treatment and recurrence rates associated with this and other yeasts. Horowiz et al. (1985) gained the impression that *Candida tropicalis* tended to be refractory and subject to recurrences. They isolated this yeast from a surprisingly high proportion, 18%, of their 99 patients with vaginal mycosis. According to the author's own experience, *Candida tropicalis* is likely to occur in only 1–3% of vaginal mycoses and does not appear to be "resistant to treatment".

These conditions should, however, be clearly distinguished from infections with *Candida glabrata* or other (rarer) facultative pathogens formerly included in the genus *Torulopsis* which may account for approx. 7–15% of vulvovaginal mycoses. The symptoms are considerably milder (Richter 1971; Lachenicht and Potel 1974; Mendling 1984).

Candida glabrata is isolated from up to 25% of healthy, asymptomatic women (Schnell et al. 1972), from 7.7% of asymptomatic pregnant women at the time of delivery (Mendling 1984) and from up to 15% of women with vaginal mycoses (Kimmig and Rieth; Mendling 1984).

The patients often have a history of slight, intermittent symptoms for a number of years, for instance, a burning sensation during coitus. The vagina appears purplish in colour and the discharge is never "typically" cheesy but rather tends to be thin and grey (but differs from that of bacterial vaginosis be being odorless). There is often no discernible increase in discharge (Fig. 126).

The examination under a phase-contrast microscope of wet-mount preparations usually shows many small oval budding cells of *Candida glabrata* or also of *Candida famata*. Occasionally the budding cells occur in the discharge in dense conglomerates whilst other blastospores seem to adhere to the vaginal epithelial cells and often appear dark under the microscope (Fig. 115 and 116). The suspected diagnosis should be confirmed by culture. On agar plates too, the yeasts tend to grow in dense "blooms". Vaginal colonization causing few symptoms does not necessarily call for treatment as the psychological effects, if the yeasts persist, can be greater than the primary symptoms.

Yeast infections of the external genital may give rise to allergic skin reactions in distant regions of the body in the forms of papules, erythema or pustules without the presence of fungi. These lesions are known as id-reactions, e.g. mycids, levurids or candidids. They can be easily missed by the gynecologist if, for instance, they take the form of a very slight scaling over the eyebrows or even if they cover the hands and forearms in a striking rash as part of a serious systemic disorder. These skin reactions disappear without intrinsic treatment after elimination of the yeasts at the sites of infection (Rieth 1979; Nolting and Fegeler 1984).

7 Diagnostic Methods

7.1 Wet-Mount Preparations

The simplest way to collect vaginal secretions is with the aid of a speculum which is drawn from the fornix vaginae over the anterior vaginal wall (Schnell 1973). Some authors object to this method because of the admixture of cervical mucus and instead recommend taking a swab of the lateral vaginal wall (Jenny, personal communication 1985). The disadvantage of this method is that the number of fungi available for examination may be much smaller (see below).

The use of a wet-mount preparation in physiological saline is unreliable (Lachenicht and Potel 1969; Seyfert 1976). No better results are achieved with wet preparations in 10-15% KOH solution or tetraethylammonium hydroxide (a method which is useful for the dissolution of keratin skin scales in dermatological examinations for fungi but not for gynecological examinations of the keratin-free vaginal epithelium) nor by the use of methylene blue, Gram's or Papanicolaou's stains (Fig. 119) (Schnell 1980).

Even in clinically obvious mycoses, the demonstration of yeasts by phase-contrast microscopy (which is preferable to standard light microscopy) (Fig. 114) is only successful in 30-90% of cases – depending on the signs and the investigator. Hantschke (1981) maintained that a fungal count of not less than 10^4/ml was required in order to obtain a positive result in a wet preparation. The total count of the vaginal mycoflora in patients with colpitis ranges from 10^3 to 10^9 fungal elements although lower counts may be associated with definite symptoms (Müller and Nold 1981). These two authors were able to show that with vaginal fungal counts of 10^4, wet preparations were positive in only 47% of cases and with counts of 10^7 in only 80%.

In the case of, for instance, *Candida albicans,* the formation of germ tubes and pseudohyphae is a condition for the transition from colonization to infection. It is therefore important for pseudohyphae to be sucessfully demonstrated in wet preparations. This is not always the case in practice. In one of our own studies involving 63 patients with vaginal mycosis caused by *Candida albicans,* the demonstration of pseudomycelia was twice as likely if the symptoms had lasted for more than one week (the isolation of pseudohyphae was always easier from scrapings of the vaginal wall than from the discharge). In total, however, they were detected in only 27 of the 63 cases (43%) with microscopic examinations lasting about 30 sec at a magnification of × 400. Budding cells alone were seen in 22 other cases (35%). This means that the microscopic tests were negative in 14 cases (22%) although cultures gave positive results (Mendling and Plempel 1982).

These figures are likely to approximate those obtained in practice and concur with most of those quoted in the literature.

The experience of individual authors who obtained positive results by means of direct microscopy in 90% of cases (Jenny 1977, 1984) must be regarded as exceptional. The resultant rejection of examination by culture is based on a failure to appreciate its diagnostic and therapeutic advantages and inhibits progress. Growing fungi in glucose solution (Jenny 1984), beer (Arabin and Malicke 1983) or Sabouraud's solution (Hain 1985) merely gives a better type of wet preparation. To identify the genus and species, culturing on agar is still indispensable.

7.2 Identification by Culture

If a direct preparation is negative, a mycological culture is indispensable to confirm the diagnosis. It is desirable even if budding cells can be demonstrated microscopically in order to identify the particular species of *Candida*. This may be of value for atypical cases and recurrences. If pseudohyphae are demonstrated, it is often possible to omit culturing in view of the present-day drive to cut costs.

It is not always necessary to carry out mycological tests to monitor clinical impressions of a therapeutic response but they are always recommended after recurrences. In such cases culture tests should be carried out for at least one week after the last topical antimycotic treatment. Wet-mount preparations alone are wholly inadequate for such cases. When using cultures to monitor the response to treatment, it should be borne in mind that residues of antifungal agents may remain in the vagina for 4 to 6 days after the last dose and may thus inhibit fungal growth on agar plates.

A number of solid and liquid culture media are available for diagnostic culture tests (Rieth 1978; Heber and Hauss 1983). Liquid media raise the yield by a few percent but solid media are wholly adequate for diagnosis under practice conditions (Gemeinhardt 1971; Schnell 1984). Culture media that have proved useful because they allow yeasts to develop their characteristic growth patterns, include Sabouraud's 2% glucose agar, Kimmig's agar (e.g. Merck) and Nervina agar according to Grütz III (Fig. 3-79, 84-87). The new Candida-II (Biotest) agar is also very sensitive and rarely encourages the growth of bacterial contaminants (Schnell 1983) but the macroscopic and microscopic appearance of the yeasts is often uncharacteristic (Fig. 68 and 95). "Selective agars" with additives of cycloheximide or other agents that inhibit the growth of bacteria or other microorganisms may also inhibit the growth of some facultatively pathogenic yeasts and thus cannot be generally recommended (Weber and Hauss 1983). They are, however, suitable for the examination of material subject to marked bacterial contamination, e.g. feces.

Nickerson's agar, popular in many countries because of the bismuth indicator that stains yeasts (but not only yeasts) brown should no longer be used; a number of bacteria commonly occurring in the vagina (e.g. E-coli, Staphylococci, Klebsiella species a.s.o.) also grow as brown colonies and 20-50% of cultures have given false positives when read by workers inexperienced in mycology (Schnell 1983). *Rhodotorula* spp. often do not form red colonies and consequently are not identified, and *Candida glabrata,* for instance, usually fails to grow at all from a relatively small but clinically possibly important inoculum (Fig. 69, 98 and 100).

The author's own investigations (in collaboration with B. Patschorke) have shown that 10 cells of *Candida albicans* per millilitre physiological saline form clearly visible colonies on Grütz III, Sabouraud's 2% dextrose agar and Candida-II agar but not on Nickerson's agar (Fig. 97). If a smear is made with a cotton wool swab from a suspension of 10^3 cells per ml, *Candida albicans* will grow on all plates but *Candida glabrata* will not grow on Nickerson's agar even at 10^4 cells/ml (Fig. 98 and 99). This means that live yeasts can be cultured on suitable media even in cases of exceedingly sparse colonization of the vagina.

Little is now heard of Microstix-Candida, a test strip which at first was welcomed by a number of workers (Vögtle-Junkert 1976; Schurz et al. 1979; Schnell 1980). In our view, its several disadvantages (complicated handling, difficulty in the microscopic evaluation of the yeast colonies and high cost) make its diagnostic usefulness inferior to that of agar plates.

It sometimes happens that a fungal culture turns out negative in a case of vaginal mycosis despite the use of a suitable agar and despite the microscopic demonstration of budding cells. In such cases, it is important to find out if the patient has used antifungal pessaries or creams from a current pack before her visit to the physician. Residues of antifungal agents may remain in the vagina for days and inhibit fungal growth.

The growth of yeasts on agar may also be wholly or partly inhibited by lubricating oils or other substances introduced into the vagina prior to cultural examination.

A morphological differentiation of established colonies on rice agar or a biochemical determination of the species by measurement of the fermentation or assimilation reactions (e.g. by API 20 C Auxanogramme) is not normally required under practice conditions but may, in individual cases, provide data to help explain persistence, sources of recurrence or a change in the pathogen. This method may also reveal multiple infections with two or more species (Rieth 1972). A reinfection may be simulated after the treatment and elimination of *Candida albicans* by the persistance of, for instance *Candida glabrata*. Such species identification may present problems despite modern facilities, even in the hands of experienced workers; sometimes strains of one species of yeast may have the same biochemical pattern and not even be morphologically distinguishable (e.g. *Candida guilliermondii* or *Candida famata*).

Any used agar plates must be correctly destroyed. This can be done by heat, i.e. autoclaving in heatproof bags, or chemically with disinfectants approved by the competent authorities (in Germany this is the Deutsche Gesellschaft für Hygiene und Mikrobiologie) (Weber and Hauss 1983).

7.3 Serological Investigations

Tests for antibodies in candidoses are solely of diagnostic value and provide no information on the immunological status of the patient (Summaries given by Müller 1972, 1974, 1978; Seeliger et al. 1974; Fasel and Seeliger 1983). As gynecological yeast infections are almost always superficial and easily accessible to clinical diagnosis and cultural examination, serological tests to confirm the diagnosis are of limited value in this field. It is only for seriously ill gynecological patients requiring interdisciplinary care that serological tests may be useful in monitoring the response.

Mycoses of the mucous membranes do not always cause significant changes in titer and the latter may be within the normal range. Commensal colonizations do not normally cause significant titers. Of the many methods such as the complement fixation test, cell agglutination, precipitation, indirect immunofluorescence test, indirect hemagglutination test and immunoelectrophoresis, the last three are of importance for the early diagnosis and monitoring of the response in mycoses in general medicine and intensive care units.

The indirect hemagglutination test using polysaccharides against glycoprotein antigens on the walls of *Candia* cells (serotype A) is suitable, by measurement of IgM, for the early diagnosis of superficial and deep candidoses as well as for monitoring patients at risk.

The indirect immunofluorescence test for the detection of IgG class antibodies is more suitable for the diagnosis and follow-up of manifest candisoses.

Immunoelectrophoresis is used to differentiate between mucosal and systemic mycoses by measurement of somatic protein antigens from inside the yeast cells. Protein antigens are released in systemic mycoses.

Other new diagnostic tests are undergoing trials and some are actually on the market, for instance, a direct enzymatic immune kit for protease antigens to detect yeast invasions in relatively deep tissue layers (Böning et al. 1986) or the latex agglutination test for the early diagnosis of deep mycoses in oncology or immunosuppressed patients (Hantschke 1986).

patients at risk (for instance an obese diabetic with carcinoma of the uterus on long-term gestagen treatment, or a very old patient about to undergo vulvectomy) should invariably be monitored at least by *cultural* diagnostic tests.

8 Therapy

It is obvious that vulvovaginal candidosis which causes pain or discomfort requires treatment. Yet whether treatment is also required for an asymptomatic vaginal yeast colonization by *Candida albicans* in a healthy individual is a matter of controversy. Therapy is always recommended during pregnancy to protect the fetus from neonatal mycosis. Since the physiological human vaginal flora does not include facultative pathogenic yeasts which may in cases of immune deficiency result in infection of the patient or her partner with candidosis, it is often recommended that the fungi be treated wherever they are found, because only this rigorous management may restrict the relatively widespread manifestation of yeasts. Other authors suggest the more pragmatic approach of only treating when there are clinical signs of infection. Considering the fact that the principal reservoir of yeast in man is the digestive tract, which is also a source of vaginal colonizing, the most important measure into achieve a reduction in human pathogenic fungi is to effect a radical change in the widespread hypercaloric carbohydrate take of people in the industrial countries. This kind of diet has led to an almost 70-fold increase in sugar consumption during the last 20 years (Rieth, Medical Tribune No. 44, 31. 10. 1986).

Without any doubt, there is no benefit from human pathogenic yeasts, and therefore even asymptomatic colonization has to be removed, at least in high-risk patients.

Rieth (1980) listed 123 substances which can be or have been used against mycoses. Numerous agents can also be used against candidoses. Nowadays people are again turning to natural cures, e. g., garlic extract which is a fungistat and fungicide (Barone and Tansey 1977; Sandhu et al. 1980).

Even today nonspecific dyes are used in dermatomycoses and occasionally in vaginal mycoses. They have the advantage of being cheap and include Pyoktanin 10% (Littauer 1923), gentian violet 2% (Sjovall 1942), and brilliant green 2% (De Palo e Papadia 1957) (quoted in Kruschwitz 1976). They are bacteriostatic, bactericidal, and mycocidal and act by means of interaction with peripheral anion groups on the cell surface, thus making reproduction impossible (Costa et al. 1987).

Disadvantages of these agents are skin pigmentation, skin intolerance, and, in the case of boric acid which is occasionally used, toxic side effects. The application of these agents only had a curing rate of 60%–70% (Kruschwitz 1976).

Hazen and Brown (1950) first isolated the tetraene antibiotic nystatin from *Streptomyces noursei*. It was the first agent discovered which is effective against yeast fungi and is very compatible; there is practically no intestinal resorption. Thus it became a popular preparation to treat vaginal candidosis and to reduce intestinal yeasts. Similar results may be reported to amphotericin B and pimaricin (natamycin). These polyene macrolide antibiotics change the permeability of the cytoplasmic membrane by forming complexes with local membrane ergosterol (Otten and Plempel 1977, Plempel 1980, Scheklakow et al. 1981). In vaginal candidosis a therapy period of 15 days was suggested, later 6 and 3 days. Due to the relatively narrow active spectrum of polyenes, their nonresorption during oral application, their intravenous toxicity, etc., it was necessary to look for new and better antimycotics.

Based on the antimycotic effect of benzimidazoles (discovered by Kimmig and Rieth in 1949), there was an intensive search for clinically suitable agents. The historical breakthrough was finally achieved by Plempel et al. (1969), when they presented clotrimazole, the first clinically suitable imidazole antimycotic which today continues to play a very important role in mycosis therapy. In recent years, additional derivatives have been clinically tested and marketed; almost all of them are applicable for vulvovaginal mycoses (Table 10).

Azole antimycotics are characterized by a higher and more rapid efficacy against fungi, and due to their simultaneous activity against staphylococci may produce a more rapid cure of superinfected vul-

Table 10. Agents used in the treatment of vulvovaginal mycoses

Nonspecific dyes:
 Crystal violet
 Gentian violet
 Brilliant green

Others:
 Boric acid (banned in Germany)
 Dequalinium chloride
 Ciclopiroxolamine
 Povidone-iodine

Established polyenes:
 Nystatin
 Amphotericin B
 Natamycin (pimaricin)

Recent Azoles

Imidazoles:
 Clotrimazole
 Miconazole nitrate
 Econazole nitrate
 Isoconazole nitrate

Triazole:
 Terconazole

Oral imidazole derivative:
 Ketoconazole
In future oral Triazole:
 Itraconazole

Unsuitable for vaginal mycoses/gynecological practice
 Flucytosine
 Griseofulvin
 Tolnaftate

val mycoses. Common features of the azole antimycotics are (Plempel 1980):

- Broad antimycotic spectrum of efficacy
- High intensity of antimycotic activity
- Partially fungicidal type of effect
- Enzyme induction and metabolism in the liver after oral application

In contrast to the effect of amphotericin on preformed membrane particles (formation of complexes with the ergosterol of the cell membrane), azoles are only effective against organisms with active cellular metabolism, because they limit the enzymatic transformation of lanosterol into ergosterol. This results in defects in the outer and inner membrane surfaces, the exit of low molecular weight cell components, and finally respiratory failure and cell death (Kern and Zimmermann 1977). This explains the fact that antimycotics have a greater efficacy during formation of germ tubes or pseudomycelium in yeast (Niimi et al. 1985).

The question of possible resistance development is often raised. We should distinguish between resistance to therapy and primary and secondary resistance to antimycotics. Therapy resistance is the result of medication and host features and is not the subject of this book. Primary resistance of pathogenic yeast to azoles has not been detected.

Yeasts are eukarionts and in contrast to bacteria (prokarionts) are not able to develop secondary resistance to a primarily effective imidazole or polyene antimycotic, because they do not possess plasmids. Bacterial plasmids are extrachromosomal DNA bodies able to transmit information about resistance. Yeasts, however, carry in their reservoir of DNA constant antimycotic sensitivity (Krempl-Lamprecht 1985), so secondary resistance may not be expected to develop in vivo. But there are reports of in vitro and in vivo resistance. In vitro resistance depends particularly on the test conditions and may be simulated by various factors, e.g., the inoculum effect (Plempel 1980).

However, some strains of *Candida albicans* in patients with chronic recurrent mucocutaneous candidosis have been described that are resistant both clinically and in vitro to some azoles (Smith et al. 1986), and furthermore are not able to bind polyenes (Hitchkock et al. 1987). It was suggested that this may partly be due to a yeast with a changed cell membrane composition, in which the ratio of phospholipids to esterified sterols is decreased, thus preventing azoles from being introduced into ergosterol metabolism. This yeast could have been a mutated laboratory species, the ergosterol of which was substituted by a variant.

Doubt was cast on these reports after precise follow-up studies

41

were done (Clissold 1987) and they were not confirmed by subsequent studies (Krempl-Lamprecht, pers. comm.). These few observations do not seem to be clinically important, and the recommendation remains valid that assessment of resistance of yeast fungi in vaginal candidoses is usually not needed. Azole antimycotics are known to have a very broad spectrum of activity, including dermatophytes, yeasts, biphasic fungi, and molds. The MIC values are usually in the range 0.1–2 µg/ml for yeasts and dermatophytes (Otten and Plempel 1977). On the other hand, the effective doses of polyenes are somewhat higher (MIC 4–16 µg/ml for nystatin and pimaricin in vitro).

Against *Candida (Torulopsis) glabrata* clotrimazole often has a MIC of 4–8 µg/ml (Otten and Plempel 1977). Ketoconazole, itraconazole, terconazole and other new azoles show under test conditions the same efficacy against *Candida glabrata* as against *C. albicans*. The general activity of new triazoles against yeasts and dermatophytes is usually higher than that of the classic imidazoles, both when measured in vitro and especially in vivo (Isaacson et al. 1985). Azoles may be antibacterial as well as having an antimycotic effect. Clotrimazole is known to be antibacterial against gram-positive cocci and *Corynebacterium minutissimum,* the pathogen of erythrasma. The MIC against streptococci and staphylococci, which commonly occur in the vulvovaginal region, ranges between 0.5 and 10 µg/ml.

The formulation of clotrimazole with lactic acid in a single-dose vaginal tablet was observed to be effective not only against fungi and gram-positive bacteria but also against gram-negative bacteria such as *Proteus, Klebsiella, E. coli,* and *Pseudomonas;* this could not be ascribed to the lactic acid alone (Schaller 1982). Efficacy against anaerobic organisms such as the *Bacteroides* species and *gardnerella vaginalis,* which are of even greater importance in gynecology than the above-mentioned aerobic pathogens, would seem likely on the basis of the MIC values of 2–16 µg/ml.

The efficacy spectrum of the imidazoles and triazoles in vitro does not include the so-called Döderlein's bacillus, which is part of the physiological vaginal flora. Careful estimations by Müller et al. (1981) showed that it is increased in vaginal candidosis, possibly because the metabolic products of the fungi provide them with particulary favorable conditions. Isoconazole treatment did not lead to a significant reduction of lactobacillae. However, Hantschke and Zabel (1979) had the impression that, in contrast to the polyene therapy, clotrimazole induced a significant temporary reduction of lactobacillae, although this was only based on estimates using gram preparations. Trichomonas vaginalis is also removed by a clotrimazol dose of 100 µg/ml, but clinically treatment of trichomoniasis is not normally with antimycotics because oral therapy is appropriate in this disease, and metronidazole is significantly more effective. For the azole antimycotics that can be administered orally such as ketoconazole and itraconazole, the MIC values in trichomoniasis are too high for effective levels to be reached.

The topical treatment of vulvovaginal candidosis by azoles generally has no significant side effects. Less important side effects are the occasionally occurring local irritations, which become noticeable as short-lasting burning sensations after application and are reported in nearly all therapy studies at a rate of 1%-10%. It has to be considered, however, whether these side effects may be caused by other agents that are contained in most galenic preparations.

Allergic reactions may occur to the dissociated constituents of yeast cells resulting from therapy. Allergic reactions to azoles may also occur and can even cause an anaphylactic shock, but this is extremely rare and is not to be expected with topical use (Raulin and Frosch 1987).

In intravaginal treatment with azoles, 3%-10% (-30%) of the active substance applied is resorbed transvaginally, the figure being dependent on the galenical and the active substances (Patzschke et al. 1976; Rindt et al. 1979; Täuber 1981). Due to their rapid metabolism in the liver the effective blood levels of these drugs are so low after vaginal resorption (Ritter et al. 1982; Kennedy and Friedmann 1985) that there is not even danger to the fetus in pregnant patients. Retrospectively, after some millions of applications during pregnancy, no connection with neonatal damage has been found.

Very good results were obtained world-wide concerning the incidence of undesired side effects of oral treatment by ketoconazole. Out of 1634 women with vaginal candidosis receiving the same short-term therapy lasting 5 days, 5.2% complained about side effects, in most cases nausea or headache. In patients with vaginal candidosis receiving 5-10 days of oral therapy, the risk of ketoconazole-induced hepatitis is said to be 1 : 500000-1 : 1000000 (Cauwenbergh 1984, 1985).

All the azoles, whether administered orally or parenterally, are contraindicated in pregnant women, as animal trials have shown maternal and fetal toxicity and teratogenity at high doses (syndactylia and cleft palate). If in early pregnancy a 5- to 10-day course of treatment is given unwittingly, and this has been at the doses normally used in treatment of vaginal mycoses, then, in our opinion (after explanation to the patient of the special risks) termination of pregnancy is not advised.

At the beginning of the 1970s the imidazoles clotrimazole, miconazole nitrate, and a little later the structurally almost identical econazole nitrate were introduced as the first azole antimycotic agents. For intravaginal therapy with miconazole a treatment length of 7-14 days was and is used, this being with miconazole similar to the suggested period for polyene preparations. For clotrimazole and econazole nitrate, 6 days of treatment were recommended. Although imidazoles can reach intracellular yeasts, it is though unlikely that there is penetration of the active substance into deep epithelium layers. Therefore, a period of treatment of at least 6 days is necessary in order that the deep-lying yeast can be brought into contact with the antimycotic through the natural estrogen-induced proliferation of vaginal epithelium, and a full cure thus be brought about.

The formulation has to be placed into the vagina as a vaginal tablet or suppository or as the cream by applicator in the evening. By means of the body warmth and vaginal moisture the drugs are dissolved within minutes or hours and are distributed in the vagina. Some of the drug is lost by discharge, the amount depending on the behavior of the patient and conditions in the vagina. This is often used as an argument against coitus during therapy, but I do not think that this prohibition is always necessary. It appears reasonable in cases of vaginal candidosis to apply the cream in the vulval and perianal regions, even if these are symptom free. Conversely, in cases of vulval candidosis the symptom-free vagina should be treated by means of vaginal suppository because in both cases yeast are always detectable at both sites.

Routine simultaneous genital treatment of the symptom-free partner is controversial, and leads to the question of whether genital candidosis should be classified as a sexually transmitted disease. In our opinion, only the recurrent genital candidosis of predisposed women is sexually transmissible. Most experts advise treating the partner simultaneously both because it is common to detect the fungus on the penis (Lachenicht and Potel 1974; Rodin and Kolator 1976) or in sperm fluid (Gilpin 1967) and because of the high rate of candidal balanitis in the partners (Raab 1978). Conversely, when treating the yeast balanitis the concurrent treatment of even symptom-free female partners is recommended (Nolting 1976; Davidson, in Robertson 1982)

The patients's compliance is an important factor in the choice of drug today (Rausch et al. 1979; Robertson 1982). At the beginning of the 1980s a vaginal tablet was first produced containing 500 mg clotrimazole and additional lactic acid, conceived as a single-dose therapy. The addition of lactic acid improved the low solubility in water thus allowing a much greater part of the active substance to be released in the vagina. Our own trials have shown that such treatment gives drug levels for a number of days that are similar to those given by doses of 100 or 200 mg each day for several days (Mendling and Plempel 1982).

The therapeutic results in treatment of acute vaginal mycosis are good for marketed azole antimycotics. Cohen (1985) compared all topical therapies for acute vaginal candidosis and demonstrated their similarity regarding mycological and clinical cure, whether using 15-, 6-, 3-, or 1-day treatment (Table 11).

In a randomized comparative study over a period of 16 years, he showed that all forms of therapy attained a cure rate of about 75%–80%. This result is similar to our own clinical experiences over 10 years; it seems to be realistic, and is a convincing argument for short-term therapy as far as acute vaginal candidosis is concerned.

As yet, the only commercially available oral imidazole antimycotic is ketoconazol. In recent years the use of ketoconazole has been wide spread in the gynecological field, both because of the impression that in some women conventional topical therapy fails, and because some women prefer oral therapy to vaginal therapy. The rec-

Table 11. Comparison of mycological response rates 35 days after treatment. Results of a 16-year study randomized within the broken lines. (Modified from Cohen 1985.)

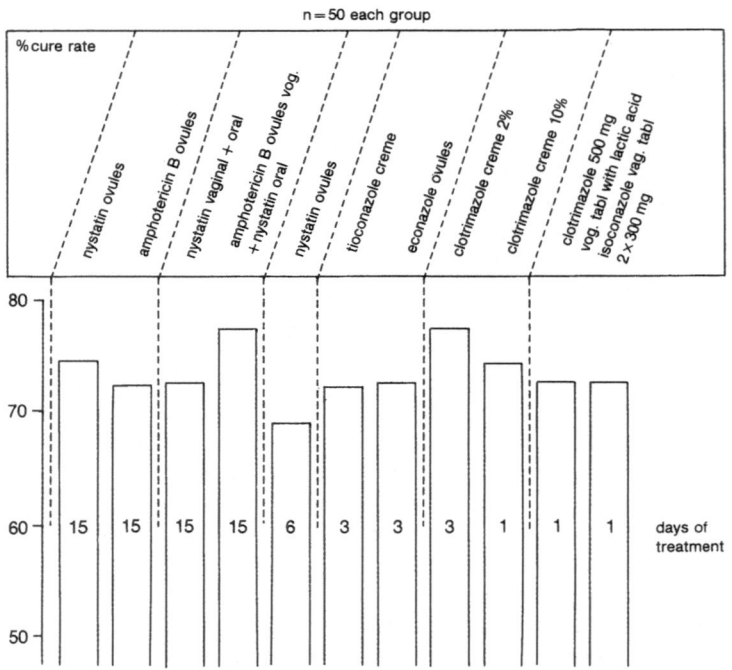

ommended form of therapy was 2 × 200 mg for 5 days. According to the literature, this treatment gives mycological cure rates of about 80%–90%, similar to the results of topical treatment (Clissold 1987). It has been shown that routine treatment with any of current antimycotics usually gives only temporary relief of symptoms after repeated and long-term application.

Various oral regimens have been tested and, especially by Sobel (1985, 1986), suggested as compromise solutions. For chronic recurrent vulvovaginal candidosis, he gave initially 400 g ketoconazole daily over 14 days, followed by a monthly intermittant therapy or prophylaxis of 400 g daily given over 5 days during menstruation.

There was a recurrence rate of 57.1% within 6 months. As an alternative they tried long-term prophylaxis with 100 mg ketonazole for 6 months daily; over a further 6 months there was a recurrence rate of 47.6%.

These results indicated that even a topical short-term treatment of only 1 day with an azole derivative may have a similar effect but with significantly less risk of problems of contraception, hepatotoxicity, and compliance.

In view of the changes from the normal distribution of T lymphocytes found in our own studies in such patients, our own therapeutic concept will in future be based on the following:

1. Controlling yeasts intravaginally using a 1-day treatment (here clotrimazole), repeated in case of recurrences
2. Attempting to influence the T lymphocyte count and the subpopulations by means of thymopentine (Mendling and Koldowsky 1987)

Permanent protection by subinhibitory and therefore very low nontoxic oral doses of azole is also plausible and should be tested, because it was shown that yeast cells thus treated in vivo lost their pathogenic efficacy (Plempel and Berg 1984). So far there is no strong argument for oral treatment of vaginal candidosis, particularly since in these mostly young women secure contraception must be taken into consideration. From our own investigations, however, oral treatment has a greater efficacy in recurrent vaginal candidosis when the patient has and wishes to keep an intrauterine device (IUD). Budding cells seem to reach more proximal parts of the cervical canal along the thread of the IUD, thus acting as a source of recurrent infections in predisposed women if topical antimycotics are not able to reach them there. The domain of ketoconazole in gynecology at present is in the treatment of chronic recurrent candidosis, as well as in special cases of vulvovaginal candidosis in patients in whom vaginal suppositories or cream may not be applied optimally.

Recurrent chronic vaginal mycosis, which often recurs each month, usually premenstrually, and can remain for years, occurs in 1%–5% of cases. It is thus relatively infrequent but is a particular burden for patients and physicians (Ludwig et al. 1969; Hurley 1975). Predisposing endogenous and exogenous factors should be eliminated as far as possible before specific therapy is terminated.

The various therapeutic possibilities available to date in such patients are an expression of helplessness and cannot be convincing because of the absence of effective cure. This cannot be attributed to a failure of the effective antimycotics, but to the predisposing factors in the infected patients and the difficulty of keeping new yeasts from them.

With this treatment at least freedom from symptoms may be attained, in these patients, even though no causal therapy of the cellular defense is yet possible.

The vaginal complaints caused by *Candida (Torulopsis) glabrata* are mostly not severe. Some patients are made aware of their slight discharge or occasional burning sensation by the gynecologist who has detected yeast in the vaginal secretions (mostly masses of them) and who asks in a suggestive manner about symptoms. In our opinion, which has changed with time, generally healthy women should only be treated if fungi can be identified in culture as *Candida glabrata* (or related facultative pathogenic species; see Table 1) and the patient has severe complaints. Unfortunately, it is quite problematic to eliminate these yeasts from the vagina with any of the currently available antimycotics. In laboratory studies the fungi are found to be sensitive to the drug, and the reasons for the persistence of the disease are as yet unknown.

That ketoconazole has no greater effect than topical azoles against fungi indicates that topical treatments should be tried first.

Here, a single-dose therapy repeated at 5-day intervals is a good choice as it causes the patient relatively little inconvenience.

In uncomplicated acute vulvovaginal candidosis, no treatment other than the specific antimycotic therapy is necessary, although treatment of the partner is usually recommended. In cases of chronic recurrent vulvovaginal candidosis, usually *Candida albicans,* all similar facultative pathogenic yeasts on the skin and mucous membranes of the patient and her partner should be eliminated as long as she has not been made immune to those organisms by increasing tolerance (T lymphocytes). Because of the great quantity of similar yeast in the digestive tract (Blaschke-Hellmessen 1979; Odds 1979; Meinhof 1982) it is recommended that these be reduced as much as

Table 12. Symptoms, courses and treatments of vulvovaginal mycoses

Pathogen	*Candida albicans*	*Candida glabrata (Torulopsis* and related species)	Other *Candida* spp. (apart from those known formerly as *Torulopsis* spp.
Symptoms	Start normally acute with itching and burning redness of the vagina, copious yellowish-white discharge; vulvitis common;	Few symptoms: occasionally mild burning, vagina barely reddened, if anything livid, sparse thin, pale grey discharge, vulvitis rare.	Similar to *Candida albicans*
Course	Short and violent, chronic recurrences are rare but present problems when they do arise.	Usually chronic over weeks or years	Similar to *Candida albicans?*
Treatment	Topically with imidazoles or polyenes, 1-day treatment with imidazoles; in case of recurrence in patients with IUD, oral ketoconazole for 5–10 days.	Difficult: systematically for not less than 2 weeks with amphotericin B or topically with imidazoles	Similar to *Candida albicans?*

Elimination of yeasts from the alimentary tract, prophylaxis on re-exposure and treatment of sexual partner recommended in the case of recurrences. Abstinence from sexual intercourse is unnecessary with any treatment.

Chronic recurrent vaginal mycosis (e.g. 3 times within 6 months): If correct topical therapy, treatment of the sexual partner and elimination of yeasts from carriage sites have proved inadequate and there is no discernible or no treatable basic illness, we recommend a compromise solution of a topical one-dose treatment with an imidazole before the symptoms (usually premenstrual) manifest themselves; repeat, if required, after 6 days (objective: freedom from symptoms where it is not possible to eliminate the fungi). Future aim: To strengthen the body's defense system.

Resistance to polyenes or imidazoles:	None known.		

possible using the intestinally unresorbable polyene antimycotics. However, the yeasts in the intestine cannot be completely destroyed. In the long term, success may be attained by reducing intestinal sugar and carbohydrate supply and by promoting the thorough cleansing of the intestine by roughage-rich vegetable foodstuffs (Rieth 1984, 1985). Due to intestinal resorption ketoconazole is not suitable for clearing the intestinal contents sufficiently of yeasts. Bladder mycosis is extremely rare. Finding yeast in mid-stream or catheter urine in women with vaginal mycosis does not indicate that there has been colonization of the bladder. These yeasts are more likely to originate in the distal vulval urethra.

The prophylaxis of neonatal mycosis is discussed in chap. 4 (p. 18).

9 Outlook

Gynecologists in hospital and practice are confronted daily with vaginal mycoses. The microscopic and cultural diagnosis is generally - if certain rules are observed - easy to learn. These measures should be a matter of course for gynecologists in order to continue to relate to the clinical case and to avoid the risk of therapeutic polypragmatism. Mycological seminars for gynecologists serve the demand for better qualifications. It is, however, unbearable that a competent physician is measured in Germany by the Kassenärztliche Vereinigung on the basis of the statistically calculated "mean value" of all his diagnostically active colleagues. If he infringes such "guide-lines" he is asked to attend a disciplinary hearing "where these measures are centered on the remarkable differences in the knowledge of the investigating physicians in the field of mycology" (Klehr 1986).

It appears that a therapeutic peak has been reached with the most potent antifungal agents that are currently on the market. Sobel (1984) was correct in expressing his disappointment when he stated that patients presenting with chronic recurrent vaginal mycoses caused by *Candida albicans* frequently failed to exhibit the risk factors constantly reiterated in the literature. Needless to say, the latter do exist but most of the affected women have the appearance of rude health and they do not suffer from diabetes, or from iron deficiency, and they are not being treated with antibiotics. Where then is their individual weakness?

Stress and other psychological phenomena have been cited as causes of vaginal mycoses and are claimed to produce reciprocal effects (Robertson 1982). It is quite conceivable that psychological factors may give rise to hormonal or immunological dysregulations and thus may be predisposing factors for vaginal mycoses.

In such cases, the gynecologist will be forced to admit that he does not yet know the whole nature of this disease and that all previous assumptions concerning predisposition and sources of recurrence are merely stations on the road to knowledge.

A therapeutic breakthrough applicable to problem cases will probably have to await new knowledge and treatments in the field of immunology. No unequivocal therapeutic successes due to activation of cell-mediated defense have so far been published. Meanwhile the author's own investigations in chronic recurrent vaginal candidoses suggest that *Candida albicans* serotype B is frequently involved and that patients tend to have a reduced total T lymphocyte count as well as characteristic changes in the interrelations of various subpopulations.

Limited experience with *Candida* antigens (Palacios 1976; Tomšíková et al. 1984), or transfer factor (Grob and Wüthrich 1974; Benz et al. 1977) and with desensibilisation (Kudelko 1971; Rosedale and Browne 1979) in the treatment of acute and recurrent vaginal mycoses suggest that lasting results may be achieved in some patients.

In the future, attention will have to center on research into cell-mediated and humoral immune defense mechanisms and their causes [Zinc deficiency? (Edman et al. 1986)], the importance of the female sex hormones and hormone receptors for yeasts, and on the interactions – if any – between cell-mediated defense and antifungal agents (Ryley 1986).

It would thus seem that even in the future, this ancient disorder will not only continue to be a disease full of riddles for the layman but remain in constant challenge for practice and research.

10 References

Adetumbi O (1984) Garlic extract exhibits antifugal activity. (Annual Meeting of the American Society for Microbiology). Mycol Observ 4 (4): 8

Anderson ML, Odds FC (1985) Adherence of *Candica albicans* to vaginal epithelia: Significance of morphological form and effect of ketoconazole. Mykosen 28: 531

Arabin H, Malicke H (1983) "mykorapid" - mykologische Schnelldiagnostik in der Gynäkologie, GIT-Suppl 3: 61

Auger P, Péloquin S, July J, Montplaisir S, Marquis G (1984) Relationship between serotype, sensitivity to ketoconazole and inhibition of pseudomycelial growth on *Candida albicans*. Mykosen 27: 498

Barone FE, Tansey MR (1977) Isolation, purification, identification, synthesis and kinetics of activity of the anticandidal Component of Allium Sativum, and a hypothesis for its mode of action. Mycologia 69: 793

Barnett JA, Payne RW, Yarrow D (1986) Yeasts - characteristics and identification. Cambridge University Press

Begemann C, Splanemann V (1986) Nektarhefen humanpathogen? Pilzdialog 2: 35

Benham RW, Hopkins AM (1933) Yeastlike Fungi Found on the Skin and the Intestinum of Normal Subjects. Arch Dermatol 28: 532

Benz CC, Thomas JW, Mandl M, Morgan N (1977) Acquired chronic candidiasis treated with transfer factor. Br J Dermatol 97: 87

Birnbaum H, Kraußold E (1975) Häufigkeit von Sproßpilz- und Trichomonaden-Infektionen bei Anwendung hormonaler und intrauteriner Kontrazeption. Zbl Gynäkol 97: 1636

Blank F, Chin O, Just G, Meranze DR, Shimkin MB, Wieder R (1968) Carcinogens from fungi pathogenic for man. Cancer Research 28: 2276

Blaschke-Hellmessen R (1968) Epidemiologische Untersuchungen zum Vorkommen von Hefepilzbei Kindern und deren Müttern. Mykosen 11: 611

Blaschke-Hellmessen R (1972) Experimentelle Untersuchungen zur Epidemiologie der Hefepilzerkrankungen bei Säuglingen und Kleinkindern. Mykosen 15: 23

Blaschke-Hellmessen R, Seebacher C, Eilmes H (1979) Vaginaler, oraler und rektaler Sproßpilzbefall bei jungen Frauen unter besonderer Berücksichtigung der Promiskuität. Zbl. Gynäkol 101: 921

Bönning B (1986) Diagnostik der tiefen Candida-Mykose mittels Enzym-immuntest auf Candida-Protease und immunhistochemischer Nachweis der Protease bei verschiedenen Manifestationen der Mykose. 20. Wiss Tagg Deutschspr Mykol Ges, Kurzfassungen

Brandt G (1984) Peripartale Candidasepsis unter dem klinischen Bild einer Listeriose. Pilzdialog 2: 19

Broschinski L, Diener W, Fischer G, Namasch KA, Wettig K, Gemeinhardt H (1986) Untersuchungen zum Vorkommen von *Candida albicans* im menschlichen Speichel in Beziehung zum Nitrat- und Nitritgehalt. Mykosen 29 (4): 177

Carlson S, Husmann KH (1956) Über die pathogenetische Bedeutung und Ausbreitung der Hefen unter der Antibiotica-Therapie. Zentralbl Bakt J Ref 160: 173

Carroll CJ, Hurley R, Stanley VD (1973) Criteria for diagnosis of Candida vulvovaginitis in pregnant women. J Obstet Gynecol Br Commonw 80: 258

Cauwenbergh G (1984) Ketoconazole, international experience in vaginal candidosis: a review. In Eliot (Ed) Oral therapy in vaginal candidosis. The Medicine Publishing Society Manchester

Cauwenbergh G (1985) International experience with ketoconazole in dermatomycoses. In: Meinhof (Ed) Oral therapy in dermatomycoses: a step forword. The Medicine Publishing Society Manchester

Clissold SP (1987) Clinical Experience in superficial Fungus Infections. In: Jones HE (Ed) Ketoconazole today. A review of clinical experience. ADIS Press Ltd Manchester

Cohen L (1985) Is more than one application of an antifungal necessary in the treatment of acute vaginal candidiasis? Am J Obstet Gynecol 152 (7): 961

Costa AL, Valenti A, Ruggeri P (1987) Effects of two stains on Blastoconidia of Candida albicans: Scanning Electron Microscope Studies. Mycosen 30: 69

Cran S, Dewist S, Clumeck N (1985) Fungal Infections in AIDS Patients. 2nd Eur Congr Clin Microbiol 1.–5.9. Brighton, England. Abstracts 17/4

Csángó (Ed) (1982) First International Conference on Vaginosis. Scand J Infect Dis, Suppl 40

Daschner F (1984) Bakterielle Erreger von Krankenhaus-Infektionen. Immun Infekt 12: 139

Davidson F, Oates JK (1985) The Pill does not cause "thrush". Br J Obstet Gynecol 92: 1265

Dermoumi H (1980) Resistenzbestimmung bei klinisch bedeutsamen Sproßpilzen – ein Vergleich zwischen Reihenverdünnungs- und Hemmhoftest. Mykosen 23: 1

Dermoumi H (1981) Antimykotika-Empfindlichkeit bei klinisch bedeutsamen Hefen und Schimmelpilzen im Hemmhoftest. Mykosen 25: 109

Dewhurst J (1980) Practical Pediatric and adolescent Gynecology. Marcel Dekker Inc, New York Basel

Diamond RD, Krzesicki R, Wellington J (1978) Damage to Pseudohyphal Forms of Candida albicans by Neutrophils in the Absence of Serum in vitro. J Clin Invest 61: 349

Di Menna ME (1954) Non pathogenic yeasts of the human skin and alimentary tract. A comparative survey. J Path Bact 68: 89

Dukes CD, Tettenbaum JS (1981) Studies on the potentiation of monilial and staphylococcal infection by tetracycline. In: Gardner HL, Kaufman RG (eds) Benign Diseases of the Vulva and Vagina. Second Edition. GK Hall Medical Publishers, Boston, Massachusetts

Edman J, Sobel JD, Taylor ML (1986) Zinc status in women with recurrent vulvavaginal candidiasis. Am J Obstet Gynecol 155: 1082

Effendy J, Schirrmeister U (1985) Mykologische Untersuchungen in den öffentlichen Schwimmbädern und Saunen von Marburg. Mykosen 28: 439

Eng RHK, Drehmel R, Smith SM, Goldstein EJC (1984) *Saccharomyces cerevisiae* infections in man. Sabouraudia 22: 403

Epstein B (1924) Studien zur Soorkrankheit. Jb Kinderheilk 104: 128

Farid A, Atia M, Hassonna N (1980) Production of Phosphatase Enzymes by Different Candida Species. Mckosen 23: 640

Farkas B, Simon N (1980) Der Einfluß von Antiandrogenen auf die Entstehung von vaginaler Candidosen. Mykosen 24: 203

Farrell SM, Hawkins DF, Ryder TA (1983) Scanning Electron Microscope study of *Candida albicans* Invasion of cultural Human cervical Epithelial cells. Sabouraudia 21: 251

Fasel J, Seeliger HPR (1983) Serodiagnostik der Candida-Infektionen. Mykosen 26: 109

Fegeler K, Macher E, Nolting S (1978) Tierexperimentelle Untersuchungen zur Immunität bei der Infektion mit *Candia albicans*. Mykosen 21: 127

Fegeler W, van Husen N, Witting Ch (1983) Mykologische Befunde bei Gastroskopiepatienten – Möglichkeiten einer differenzierten Bewertung. Mykosen 26: 82

Ferrante A, Tong YH (1979) Activation of the Alternative Complement Pathway by *Torulopsis glabrata*. Scand J Infect Dis 11: 77

Gardner HL, Kaufmann RH (1981) Benign Diseases of the Vulva and Vagina. GK Hall Medical Publishers, Boston, Massachusetts

Gauwerky J, Schmidt W, Kühn H, Kubli F (1983) Der vorzeitige Blasensprung: Falldarstellung einer schweren intrauterinen Pilzinfektion. Geburtsh u Frauenheilk 43: 174

Gedek B (1980) Kompendium der medizinischen Mykologie. Verlag Paul Parey, Berlin Hamburg

Gemeinhardt H (1971) Ergebnisse von kulturellen Vaginalabstrichuntersuchungen zum Nachweis von pathogenen Sproßpilzen. Dtsch Gesundh Wes 16: 1330

Gemeinhardt H (1971) Vergleich der grobquantitativen Primärkultur mit der Anreicherungskultur bei mykologischen Vaginalabstrichuntersuchungen. Z ges Hyg Grenzgeb 17: 525

Ghannoum MA, Al-Khars A (1984) Antineoplastic Agents on the Growth and Ultrastructure of *Candia albicans*. Mykosen 27: 452

Gilpin CA (1967) Resistant monilial vaginitis: the male aspect. Florida State Med J 54: 337

Göttlicher S, Madjarić J (1983) Bedeutet die orale Kontrazeption eine erhöhte Gefahr für vaginale Sproßpilzinfektionen? extracta gynäkol 7 (6): 622

Grimmer H (1968) Vulvitis (Vulvovaginitis) Candidomycetica. Z Haut- und Geschl Kr 43: 45

Grimmer H (1969) Histologischer Bildbericht Nr.217: Pilzerkrankungen des äußeren weiblichen Genitale (außer Candidiasis) – zur Klassifizierung der hautpathogenen Pilze. Z Haut- und Geschl Kr 44: 37

Grob PJ, Wüthrich B (1974) Transfer factor therapy in a patient with chronic vaginal candidiasis. J Obstet Gynecol Br Commonw 81: 812

Hain K (1985) Hefediagnostik im "Fallpunkte-Labor". GIT Suppl 5: 70

Hantschke D, Zabel M (1979) Das Verhalten der physiologischen Vaginalflora während antimykotischer Therapie. Mykosen 22: 267

Hantschke D (1981) Notwendige und mögliche Laboruntersuchungen in der gynäkologischen Praxis bei Verdacht auf Vaginalmykose. In: Seeliger HPR (Hrsg) Gyno-Travogen-Monographie

Hantschke D (1986) Candida-Antigennachweis – Fortschritt in der Diagnostik von Endomykosen. 20.Wiss Tagg Deutschspr Mykol Gesellsch, Kurzfassungen

Hasenclever F, Mitchel WO (1961) Antigenic Studies of Candida. J Bacteriol 82: 570

Hauck H, Simon M, Simon B, Geschwender B, Djawari D (1985) Beeinflußbarkeit von Phagozytose und intrazellulärer Abtötung von Candida albicans durch PMNL durch Stammeigenschaften dieses Erregers. Zbl Haut- u Geschlechtskr 150: 660

Haussmann D (1870) Die Parasiten der weiblichen Geschlechtsorgane des Menschen und einiger Tiere. Verlag August Hirschwald, Berlin

Hazen EL, Brown R (1950) Two Antifungal Agents Produced by a Soil Actinomycete. Science 112: 423

Heber W, Reinel D, Vogel W (1975) Hefebefunde bei Reihenuntersuchungen an Soldaten der Bundeswehr. Mykosen 18: 397

Heber W, Hauss H (1983) Mykologische Techniken in der ärztlichen Praxis. Schwarzeck Verlag, München

Heinz M, Hoyme S (1974) Gynäkologie des Kindes- und Jugendalters. 2. überarbeitete Auflage. F Enke Verlag, Stuttgart

Heite HJ, Buck A, Lehmann Ch (1964) Quantitative Untersuchungen der fungistatischen Aktivität menschlichen Serums gegen *Candida albicans*. Dermatologica 128: 350

Hildick-Smith G, Blank H, Sarkany J (1964) Fungus Diseases and their Treatment. Little Brown and Company, Boston

Hitchkock CA, Barrett-Bee KJ, Russell NJ (1987) The lipid composition and permeability to azole of an azole- and polyene-resistant mutant of Candida albicans. J Med Veter Mcol 25: 29

Hobbs JR, Bridgen D, Davidson F, Kahan M, Oates JK (1977) Immunological Aspects of Candidal Vaginitis. Proc Roy Soc Med 70: 11

Holthoff J, Blaschke-Hellmessen R, Böttger D (1976) Zur Problematik der Vaginalmykosen in der Schwangerschaft unter besonderer Berücksichtigung des Neugeborenen. Dt Gesundh-Wesen 31: 973

Horowiz BJ, Edelstein SW, Lippman L (1985) *Candida tropicalis* Vulvovaginitis. Obstet Gynecol 66: 229

Huber A (1977) Vulvovaginitis bei Kindern und Jugendlichen. Gynäk Praxis 1: 325

Huhn FO, Stock G (1977) Bericht über eine Fadenpilz-Granulomatose der Mamma als differentialdiagnostischer Beitrag zum Bild eines "inflammatorischen Karzinoms". Geburtsh u Frauenheilk 37: 692

Hurley R (1975) Inveterate vaginal thrush. Practitioner 215: 753

Isaacson DM, Foleno B, Tolman EL, Rosenthale ME (1985) In vitro studies with Terconazole. Gynäk Rdsch 25 Suppl 1: 12

Jankowski RP, Aikins HE, Vehrson H, Gupta KG (1977) Antibacterial Activity of Amniotic Fluid against *Staphylococcus aureus, Candida albicans* and Brucella abortus. Arch Gynaecol 222: 275

Jenny J (1977) Die Phasenkontrastmikroskopie in der täglichen Praxis. Leitfaden und Bildatlas. Verlag Jenny und Artusi, Schaffhausen

Jenny J (1984) Häufigkeit und klinische Bedeutung der im Vaginalbereich vorkommenden Pilzarten. Schweiz Rundschau Med (Praxis) 73: 197

Jirovec O, Peter R, Malek J (1948) Neue Klassifikation der Vaginalbiocoenosen auf sechs Grundbildern. Gynaecologia (Basel) 126: 77

Kennedy BK, Friedmann N (1985) Terconazole Cream and Suppositories: Plasma Terconazole following vaginal Administration. Gynäk Rdsch 25 Suppl 1: 26

Kern R, Zimmermann FK (1977) Über den Wirkungsmechanismus des Antimyzetikums Econazol. Mykosen 20: 133

Kimmig J, Rieth H (1949) Die Behandlung der Dermatophyten mit neuen pilzabtötenden Verbindungen. Arch Derm Syph (Berl) 189: 265

Kimmig J, Rieth H (1961) Mykosen und Trichomonaden. Arch Gynäk 195: 31

Kimura LH, Pearsall NN (1980) Relationship between germination of *Candida albicans* and increased adherence to human buccal epithelial c... Infect Immun 28: 464

King RD, Lee JC, Morris AL (1980) Adherence of *Candida albican...* other Candida Species to Mucosal Epithelial Cells. Infect Immun 2...

Kintzel HW, Hinkel GK, Blaschke-Hellmessen R (1971) Durch *Can... bicans* und andere Hefepilze verunreinigte Frauenmilch als Ursa... Gruppeninfektionen von Frühgeborenen. Acta Paediatr Acad S... 12: 121

Klehr NW (1986) 5 Jahre Erfahrungen mit der mykologischen Dia... der Kassenarztpraxis (unter Berücksichtigung der Prüfgremie... Tagg Deutschspr Mykol Gesellsch, Kurzfassungen

Klein RS, Harris CA, Small CB, Moll B, Lesser M, Friedland...

Oral Candidiasis in high risk patients as the initial manifestation of the acquired immunodificiency syndrome. N Engl J Med 311: 354

Knippenberger H, Vanslow H, Barth H, Scheffzyk HD, Rüttgers H (1979) Sproßpilzepidemiologie an 1000 Patientinnen. Geburtsh u Frauenheilk 39: 676

Koch Y, Koch HA (1981) Zur Epidemiologie der Candidosen des Mund-Pharynx-Raumes. Mykosen 24: 197

Körte C, Schmidt P, Rieth H (1968) Wandert "Bäckerhefe" durch die intakte Darmwand? Experimenteller Beitrag zur Frage der Persorption lebender Hefen. Mykosen 11: 912

Kozinn PhJ, Taschdjian CL, Goldberg PK, Wise GJ, Toni EF, Seelig MS (1978) Advances in the Diagnosis of Renal Candidiasis. J Urol 119: 184

Krause W, Matheis H, Wulf K (1969) Experimentelle Fungiämie und Fungiurie durch orale Verabreichung großer Mengen von Candida albicans beim gesunden Menschen (Selbstversuch). Arzneim Forsch (Drug Res) 19: 85

Kreger-van Rij NJW (ed) (1984) The yeasts. A taxonomic study. Third revised and enlarged edition. Elsevier Science Publishers BV, Amsterdam

Krempl-Lamprecht L (1985) Resistenzprüfung bei Hefen – ja oder nein? Pilzdialog 3: 41

Kruschwitz S (1976) Entwicklung der Therapie der Vaginalmykosen. Dt Gesundh-Wesen 31: 970

Kudelko NM (1971) Allergy in Chronic Monilial Vaginitis. Ann Allergy 29: 266

Kuttin ES, Müller J, Melchinger H, Jaeger R (1984) Electronmicroscopic Studies of Candida albicans Infected Kidneys in Non-Immunized and Immunized Hosts. Mykosen 27: 72

ᵞhenicht Ph, Potel J (1974) Untersuchungen zur lokalen Chemotherapie d zur Epidemiologie der weiblichen Genitalmykose. I. Mitteilung: italmykose. II. Mitteilung: Epidemiologie. Arzneim Forsch (Drug ⁷4: 525 u 529

t Ph, Potel J (1976) Nachweismethoden für Hefen im Urin und sche Bedeutung. Münch med Wschr 118 Suppl 1: 43

h, Potel J, Ziegler HK (1976) Die Zervix – ein Hefereservoir? Wschr 118 Suppl 1: 39

Premenarchal Vaginitis. Obstet Gynecol 13: 723

Hefen in der Urologie. Notabene medici 8: 313

Die Therapie der Urogenitalmykose der Frau. Notabene

Candidainfektion der Harnblase. Aktuelle Urologie 5:

985) Menstruation: Tampon oder Binde? Ihre Pawählen! Ärztl. Praxis 37 (Nr 16): 598

easts. A taxonomic study. Second revised and lland Publishing Company, Amsterdam Lon-

Leoffler W (1983) Terminologie der Humanmykosen. Mykosen 26 (7): 346

Louria DB, Brayton RG (1964) A Substance in Blood Lethal for *Candida albicans*. Nature 201: 309

Ludwig AO, Murowski BJ, Sturgis SH (1969) Psychological Aspects of Gynecological Disorders. Harvard Unversity Press, Cambridge, Massachusetts

Luger A (1982) Genitale Kontaktinfektionen. G Thieme Verlag, Stuttgart New York

Malicke H (1980) Langzeitstudie über die Rezidivhäufigkeit der Vaginalmykose bei Frauen nach einfacher Lokalbehandlung des Genitales und nach zusätzlicher Lokalbehandlung des Magen-Darm-Traktes. Notabene medici 10: 164

Mathur S, Koistinen GV, Horger III E, Mahvi TA, Fundenberg H (1977) Humoral immunity in Vaginal Candidiasis. Infect Immun 15: 287

Mayer L (1862) Über die pflanzlichen Parasiten der weiblichen Sexualorgane in ihrer praktischen Bedeutung. Monatsschr f Geburtskunde u Frauenkrankheiten S 2, Verlag August Hirschwald, Berlin

Meech RJ, Smith JMB, Chew T (1985) Pathogenic mechanisms in recurrent genital candidosis in women. NZ Med J 98: 1

Meinhof W (1974) Die Salzsäure-Toleranz von Candida albicans. Mykosen 17 (12): 339

Meinhof W, Laschka P, Scherwitz Ch (1975) Ein vollsynthetisches Medium für die rasche Chlamydosporenbildung von *Candida albicans*. Mykosen 18: 291

Meinhof W (1976) Diskussions-Bemerkungen zum Vortrag von Ph Lachenicht: Pilzreservoir Zervikalkanal? Münch med Wschr 118: 60

Meinhof W (1977) Systemische Mykosen. Fortschr Med 95: 771

Meinhof W (1982) Demonstration of Typical Features of Individual *Candida albicans* Strains as a Means of Studying Sources of Infection. Chemother 28: 51

Meisels A (1969) Dysplasia and Carcinoma of the Uterine Cervix. IV. A Correlated Cytologic and Histologic Study with Special Emphasis on Vaginal Microbiology. Acta Cytol Vol 13 Nr. 4: 224

Melchinger H, Müller J, Takamiya H, Nold B (1980) Immunelektronmikroskopische Untersuchungen an Asteroid Bodies in Vaginalmaterial von Candida-Kolpitis-Patientinnen. Mykosen 23: 161

Mendling W, Haller I (1977) Zur Wirkung therapeutischer Dosen von γ-Strahlen auf *Candia albicans-Zellen* in vitro. Geburtsh u Frauenheilk 37: 947

Mendling W, Schnell JD, Spiecker R (1979) Der Einfluß der Radium-Kontaktbestrahlung auf den vaginalen Hefebefall. Geburtsh u Frauenheilk 39: 1017

Mendling W, Janssen K (1981) Drei Tage gegen die Vulvovaginalcandidose. Sexualmed 12: 471

Mendling W, Plempel M (1982) Demonstration of pseudomycelia in the vagina, yeast infection of the rectum, and one-day therapy of vaginal candidiasis. X[th] World Congress of Gynecology and Obstetrics Oct 17–22, San Francisco. Abstracs 1703

Mendling W, Plempel M (1982) Vaginal Secretion Levels after 6 Days, 3 Days and 1 Day of Treatment with 100, 200 and 500 mg Vaginal Tablets of Clotrimazole and their Therapeutic Efficacy. Chemother 28, Suppl 1: 43

Mendling W, Schnell JD (1984) Antepartale vaginale Hefekontamination heute. Mykosen 27 (11): 573

Mendling W (1984) Die Torulopsidose in der Frauenheilkunde. Geburtsh u Frauenheilk 44: 583

Mendling W (1985) Mykosen in Gynäkologie und Geburtshilfe - eine ständige Herausforderung. Gynäkologe 18 (3): 177

Mendling W, Koldovsky U (1987) T-Lymphozyten und ihre Subpopulationen bei Patientinnen mit akuter und chronisch-rezidivierender Vulvovaginalcandidose sowie erste Therapieversuche mit Timunox[R]. 21. Wiss Tagg d Deutschspr Mykol Ges, Abstracts

Monif GRG (1985) Classification and pathogenesis of vulvovaginal candidiasis. Am J Obstet Gynecol 152 (7): 935

Müller HL, Kirchhoff G (1969) Serologische Typen von *Candida albicans*. Zentralbl Bakteriol Parasitenk Infektionskr Hyg Abt 1: Orig Reihe A 210: 114

Müller HL (1972) Die Serologie der Candida-Infektionen. Klin Wschr 50: 809

Müller HL (1980) Prüfung der Keimschlauchbildung und anderer zellmorphologischer Kriterien der Sproßpilze auf einem chemisch-definierten Agar-Medium nach Wickerham (Mycoplate MA ⟨Roche⟩). Mykosen 23 (11): 609

Müller J, Nold B (1981) Quantitative Aspekte der vaginalen Mykoflora und ihre Beziehung zur klinischen Symptomatik bei Kolpitis-Patientinnen. In: Seeliger HPR (Hrsg) Gyno-Travogen-Monographie. Excerpta Medica

Müller J, Nold B, Kubitza D, Baumert J (1981) Quantitative Untersuchungen über die Döderlein-Flora gesunder sowie mykosekranker Probandinnen unter lokaler Isoconazolnitrat-Therapie. In: Seeliger HPR (Hrsg) Gyno-Travogen-Monographie. Excerpta Medica, Amsterdam Oxford Princeton

Nanjappa Chetty G, Senthamil Selvi G, Kamalam A, Thambiah AS (1980) Candidosis in Mother and Child. Mykosen 23: 580

Neumann G, Kaben U (1971) Einfluß von Östriol, Östradiobenzoat, Progesteron, Lochialsekret und Fruchtwasser auf das Wachstum von Hefepilzen in vitro. Zbl Gynäkol 93: 1147

Nickerson WJ, Irving R, Mehmert HS (1945) Sandals and hygiene and infection of the feet. Arch Dermatol Symphilol 52: 365

Niimi M, Kamiyama A, Tokunaga M, Nakayama H (1985) Germ tube - forming cells of Candida albicans are more susceptible to clotrimazole-induced killing than yeast cells. Sabouraudia: J Med Veter Mycol 23: 63

Nolting S (1976) Die Bedeutung der Candida-Vulvovaginitis und -Balanitis unter spezieller Berücksichtigung der Partnerbehandlung. Münch med Wschr 118, Supp 1: 81

Nolting S, Hagemeier H, Fegeler K (1982) Effekt von Insulin auf die Keimschlauch- und Myzelbildung von *Candia albicans*. Mykosen 25: 36

Nolting S, Fegeler K (1984) Medizinische Mykologie. Zweite, korrigierte Auflage. Springer Verlag, Berlin Heidelberg New York Tokyo

Odds FC (1979) Candida and candidosis. Leicester University Press

Oehlschlaegel G, Arweck L, Krempl-Lamprecht L (1985) Untersuchungen über die Hefeflora auf gesunder Haut. Mykosen 28: 43

Opri F (1982) Mammary mycosis. Chemotherapy 28 (Supp 1): 61

Otten H, Plempel M, Siegenthaler W (1977) Antibiotika-Fibel. G Thieme Verlag, Stuttgart

Owusu KA, Müller J, Nold B (1978) Der diagnostische Wert von Sproßpilz-Keimzahlbestimmungen im Urin. 14. Wiss Tagg d Deutschspr Mykol Ges, Abstracts

Palacios HJ (1976) Hypersensitivity as a Cause of Dermatologic and Vaginal Moniliasis Resistent to Topical Therapy. Ann Allergy 37: 110

Patt V, Niessen M, Korte W (1972) Vaginalmykosen in der Gynäkologie und Geburtshilfe. Gynäkologe 5: 217

Patt V, Korte W (1975) Vaginalmykosen. In: Hartung J, Lubach D (Hrsg) Mykosen. G Thieme Verlag, Stuttgart

Patzschke K, Wegner LA, Oberste-Lehn H, Horster FA (1976) Pharmakokinetische Untersuchungen nach topischer Anwendung von Clotrimazol (Canesten[R]). Münch Med Wschr 118 Suppl 1: 12

Petersen EE (1985) Die Aminkolpitis. Gynäkologe 18 (3): 131

Piccolella E, Lombardi G, Morelli R (1981) Generation of suppressor cells in the response of human lymphocytes to a polysaccharide from *Candida albicans*. J Immun 126: 2151

Plass ED, Hesseltine HC, Borts JH (1934) Monilia Vulvovaginitis. Am J Obstet Gynecol 21: 320

Plempel M, Bartmann K, Büchel KH, Regel E (1969) Experimentelle Befunde über ein neues, oral wirksames Antimykotikum mit breitem Wirkungsspektrum. Dtsch med Wschr 94: 356

Plempel M (1980) Pharmakokinetik der Imidazol-Antimykotika. Mykosen 23: 16

Plempel M (1986) Pilzinfektionen durch Antibiotika? FAC Fortschr antimikr antineoplast Chemother 5-3: 561

Plempel M, Berg D (1984) Reduktion der In-vivo-Virulenz von *Candida albicans* durch Vorbehandlung mit subinhibitorischen Azol-Konzentrationen in vitro. Pilze auf Haut und Schleimhaut Suppl Heft 6: 27 GIT-Verlag, Darmstadt

Preusser HJ (1982) *Trichophyton rubrum – Candida albicans*. G Fischer Verlag, Stuttgart New York

Preusser HJ, Rostek H (1983) Der Einfluß von Nährmedien und Sauerstoff-Partialdruck auf Wachstum, Morphologie und Cytologie von *Candia albicans* in vitro. Mykosen 26 (10): 501

Raab WP (1974) Pimaricin (Natamycin). G Thieme Verlag, Stuttgart

Raab W (1978) Mykosebehandlung mit Imidazolderivaten. Springer-Verlag, Berlin Heidelberg New York

Raab W, Högl F (1981) Interaktionen zwischen Polyen-Antibiotika und Imidazol-Derivaten. Mykosen 24: 65

Rätz-Günther M, Günther M, Mendling W, Schubert GE, Plempel M (1987) Prospektive mykologisch-histologische Untersuchung des Urogenitaltraktes eines unausgewählten Obduktionsgutes. 21. Wiss Tagg d Deutschspr Mykolog Ges, Abstracts

Raith L, Csató M, Dobozy A (1983) Decreased *Candida albicans* Killing Activity of Granulocytes from Patients with Diabetes mellitus. Mykosen 26: 557

Rakosi T, Nold B, Jaeger R, Müller J (1986) Immunelektronenmikroskopische Untersuchungen über pilzzellfixierte Immunglobuline in Untersuchungsmaterien von Kolpitis-Patientinnen. 20. Wiss Tagg Deutschspr Mykol Ges, Abstracts

Raulin Ch, Frosch PJ (1987) Contact Allergy to Imidazole Antimycotics. Contact Dermatitis, in Press

Rausch KD, Girardi MR, Senft HH, Korte W (1979) Vorteile der Kurzzeittherapie bei Vaginalmykosen unter sozialpsychologischen Aspekten. 9th World Congress of Gynecol and Obstetr Tokyo Oct 25-31. Abstracts

Richter K (1971) Erkrankungen der Vagina. In: Schwalm H, Döderlein G (Hrsg) Klinik der Frauenheilkunde und Geburtshilfe, Band VIII: 433 Urban u Schwarzenberg, München Berlin Wien

Richter P, Blaschke-Hellmessen R, Karntz P (1977) Häufigkeit und Bedeutung von Sproßpilzen bei Carcinoma in situ und invasivem Zervixkarzinom. Zbl Gynäkol 99: 1260

Rieth H (1967) D-H-S-Diagnostik. Fortschr Med 85: 594

Rieth H (1969) Haben Neugeborene Anspruch auf wirksame Pilzprophylaxe? Mykosen 12: 81

Rieth H (1970) Pilzerkrankungen des Urogenitaltraktes. Urologe 10: 23

Rieth H (1972) Mykologische Bildkartei, 89. Folge: Doppelinfektionen durch Hefen verschiedener Gattung und Art. Methodik und Trennung von Mischkulturen und Bedeutung der Reinzuchtstämme für die Empfindlichkeitsprüfungen gegen Antimykotika. Mykosen 15: 221

Rieth H (1978) Mykosen - Diagnose und Therapie. Hrsg: Programmed - med pharm Verlags GmbH Frankfurt/M in Zusammenhang mit dem Verband der niedergelassenen Ärzte Deutschlands e.V. Köln

Rieth H (1979) Hefe-Mykosen. Urban u Schwarzenberg, München Berlin Baltimore

Rieth H (1980) Mykosen und Antimykotika II. Teil. Pharmazie in unserer Zeit 9 Nr1

Rieth H (1984) Anti-Pilz-Diät. GIT-Suppl 6: 38

Rieth H (1984) Pilzdiagnostik - Mykosentherapie. Sammelband I-IV. Notabene medici, Melsungen

Rieth H (1985) Anti-Pilz-Diät gegen pathogene Hefen im Intestinaltrakt. pilzdialog 3: 47

Rindt W, Geibel W, Appel L (1979) Untersuchungen zur vaginalen Resorption von Econazol. Arzneim Forsch (Drug Res) 29: 697

Ritter W, Patzschke K, Krause U, Stettendorf S (1982) Pharmacokinetic Fundamentals of Vaginal Treatment with Clotrimazole. Chemother 28 Suppl 1: 37

Ritzerfeld W (1972) Entzündliche Erkrankungen der Genitalien. Bakteriologie, Virologie und Parasitologie. In: Käser O, Friedberg V, Ober KG, Thomsen K, Zander J (Hrsg) Gynäkologie und Geburtshilfe Band III. Georg Thieme Verlag, Stuttgart

Robertson WH (1982) Patient Compliance and the Short-Germ Treatment Regime. Chemother 28: 80

Robertson WH (1982) Vulvovaginal Candidiasis: Current Concepts of Diagnosis and Management. Miles Pharmaceuticals Division of Miles Laboratories, Inc USA

Rodin Ph, Kolator B (1976) Carriage of yeasts on the penis. Brit Med J I: 1123

Rodriguez M, Okagaki T, Richart RM (1972) Mycotic Endometritis Due to Candida. Obstet Gynecol 39: 292

Rosedale N, Browne K (1979) Hyposensitation in the Mangement of Recurrent Vaginal Candidiasis. Ann Allergy 43: 250

Rüther E, Rieth H, Koch H (1958) Die Bedeutung der Candidamykosen (Moniliasis) für Gynäkologie und Geburtshilfe. Geburtsh u Frauenheilk 18: 22

Ryley JF (1986) Pathogenicity of *Candida albicans* with particular reference to the vagina. J Med Veter Mycol 24: 5

Sandhu DK, Warraich MK, Singh S (1980) Sensitivity of Yeasts Isolated from Cases of Vaginitis to Aqueous Extracts of Garlic. Mykosen 23: 691

Schaller K (1982) In vitro antibacterial Activity of Different Clotrimatzole Formulations. Chemother 28 Suppl 1: 32

Scheklakow ND, Delektorski WW, Golodova OA (1980) Veränderungen der Ultrastruktur von Candida albicans unter der Einwirkung von Polyenantibiotika. Mykosen 24: 140

Scherwitz C, Rassner G (1978) Diagnostik der Candida-albicans-Mykosen in der Gynäkologie unter besonderer Berücksichtigung des Keimschlauchtests. Geburtsh u Frauenheilk 38: 53

Scherwitz C, Martin R, Ueberberg H (1978) Ultrastructural investigations of the formation of *Candida albicans* germtubes and septa. Sabouraudia 16: 115

Schnell JD, Andrews P, Plempel M (1972) Die vaginale Kontamination der weiblichen Bevölkerung einer Großstadt mit Trichomonaden und Hefen. Geburtsh u Frauenheilk 32: 1007

Schnell JD, Plempel M (1972) Penicillium im Vaginalsekret. Mykosen 15: 409

Schnell JD (1973) Zytologie und Mikrobiologie der Vagina. S Karger

Schnell JD, Voigt WH (1974) Das Verhalten von Sproßpilzen an nicht verhornendem Plattenepithel. Arch Gynäkol 217: 377

Schnell JD (1975) Soor bei Schwangeren und Neugeborenen. In: Hartung J, Lubach D (Hrsg) Mykosen. G Thieme Verlag, Stuttgart

Schnell JD (1980) Mykosen: Möglichkeiten und Grenzen der Diagnostik in der gynäkologischen Praxis. Diagnostik 13: 205

Schnell JD (1982) Vaginalmykose und perinatale Pilzinfektion. S Karger.

Schnell JD (1983) Ein neues Elektivmedium zum Hefenachweis in der gynäkologischen Praxis. 17. Wiss Tagg d Deutschspr Mykol Ges, Abstracts

Schnell JD (1986) Zur heutigen peripartalen Hefekontamination. Waren Öffentlichkeitsarbeit und moderne Antimykotika erfolgreich? 20. Wiss Tagg Deutschspr Mykol Gesellsch, Abstracts

Schurz AR, Breitfellner G, Kiesler J (1979) Die Diagnostik volvovaginaler Mykosen. Geburtsh u Frauenheilk 39: 413

Schwarze R, Blaschke-Hellmessen R, Hinkel GK, Hoffmann H, Weigl J (1976) Untersuchungen zur Soorprophylaxe Neugeborener. I. Mitteilung: Wirksamkeit einer Fungicin-(Nystatin-)Prophylaxe bei gesunden Neugeborenen. Kinderärztl Prax 7: 305

Seebacher C (1981) Zur Ätiologie und Pathogenese der Dermatitis seborrhoides infantum. Mykosen 24: 209

Scientific American (1981) 11

Seelig MS (1966) Mechanism by which antibiotics increase the incidence and severity of candidiasis and alter the immunological defenses. Bacteriol Rev 30: 442

Seeliger HPR, Tomšiková A, Török J (1974) Immunologische Reaktionen durch *Candida albicans*. Mykosen 18: 51, 119, 149

Seneca H, Longo F, Peer P (1968) Candida Pyelonephritis and Candiduria: The Clinical Significance of *Candia albicans* in Urine Cultures. J Urol 100: 266

Seyfert C (1976) Die diagnostischen Möglichkeiten der Vaginalmykose in einer gynäkologischen Ambulanz. Dt Gesundh Wesen 31: 966

Smith KJ, Warnock DW, Kennedy CTC, Johnson EM, Hopwood V, van Cutsem J, vanden Bossche H (1986) Azole resistance in Candida albicans. J Med Veter Mycol 24: 133

Sobel JD, Myers PG, Kaye D, Levison ME (1981) Adherence of *Candida albicans* to Human Vaginal and Buccal Epithelial Cells. J Infect Dis 143: 76

Sobel JD (1984) Vulvovaginal Candidiasis – What we do and what we do not know. Ann Int Med 101 Nr 3: 390

Sobel JD (1985) Management of recurrent vulvavaginal candidiasis with intermittend ketoconazole prophylaxis. Obstet Gynecol 65: 435

Sobel JD (1986) Recurrent vulvovaginal candidiasis. N Engl J Med 315 (23): 1455

Somos S, Tóth E, Loibl A, Sélley D, Csontos F, Szepes E, Gróf P (1982) Vaginalinfektion und die lokale Immunantwort im Vaginalsekret. Mykosen 25: 497

Sonck CE (1978) Yeasts from vaginal discharge. Mykosen 21: 412

Spiechowicz E, Wegman-Rzucidlo D (1971) *Candida albicans* als eine der Ursachen der prothetischen Stromatopathien. Mykosen 14: 419

Spitzbart H (1980) Neue Aspekte zur Fluordiagnostik und -therapie. Zbl Gynäkol 102: 585

Staib F, Geier R (1971) Proteolysis products of *Candia albicans* as a substratum for growth of *Staphylococcus aureus*. A preliminary report. Zbl Bact Hyp I Abt Orig A 218: 374

Syverson RE, Buckley H, Gibian J, Ryan GM (1979) Cellular and Humoral Immune Status in Women with Chronic Candida vaginitis. Am J Obstet Gynecol 134: 624

Szarmach H, Malyszko E, Wrousky A (1983) Verschiedene diagnostische und epidemiologische Probleme im Verlauf der koexistierenden Candidiasis und Trichomoniasis des Urogenitaltraktes beim Menschen. Mykosen 26: 285

Täuber U (1981) Pharmakokinetische Aspekte der Einmaltherapie von Vaginalmykosen mit Isoconazolnitrat. In: Seeliger HPR (Hrsg) Gyno-Travogen Monographie. Escerpta Medica Amsterdam Oxford Princeton

Taschdjian CL, Burchill JJ, Kozinn PZ (1960) Rapid identification of *Candida albicans* by filamentation in serum and serum substitutes. Am J Clin Path 99: 212

Tatra G (1973) Über die Häufigkeit und Therapie vulvovaginaler Mykosen bei Gastarbeiterinnen. Castellania 1: 31

Terreni AA, Strohecker JS, Dowda H Jr (1986) Candida lusitaniae septicemia in a patient on extended home intravenous hyperalimentation. J Med Veter Mycol 25: 63

Tomšíková A, Novačková D (1981) Diagnostische Bedeutung des *Candida albicans* abtötenden Faktors. Mykosen 24: 677

Tomšíková A, Kotal L, Zavazal V, Seberová E, Sterba J (1984) Therapeutic effects of fungus vaccines and antisera. Tag-Ber Akad Landwirtsch Wiss DDR Berlin 222: 385

Vanbreuseghem R (1970) Post-mortem mycological investigation of 100 Cancerous patients. Mykosen 13: 337

Vandenbussche M, Swinne D (1984) Oral yeast carriage in Denture Wearers. Mykosen 27: 431

Vögtle-Junkert U (1976) Neues Hilfsmittel in der Pilzdiagnostik: Teststreifen Mikrostix®-Candida. Münch med Wschr 118: 885

Volkheimer G (1967) Zur Pathophysiologie der Dünndarm-Resorption - das Phänomen der Persorption. Akt Kongreßber 2: 61, 17. Ärztl. Fortbildungskurs Bad Kissingen

Waldman RH, Cruz JM, Rowe DS (1971) Immunglobulin Levels and Antibody to *Candida albicans* in Human Cervicovaginal Secretions. Clin exp Immunol 9: 427

Walther T, Rytter M, Schönborn C, Hanstein UF (1986) Differences in the Intracellular Killing of Proteinase-Positive and Proteinase-Negative Candida albicans Strains by Granulocytes. Mykosen 29 (4): 159

Weber A, Kolb S (1986) über die mehrmalige Isolierung von *Caudida pulch-*

errima (Lindner) Windisch aus Blutkulturen eines parenteral ernährten Patienten. Mykosen 29: 127

Wegmann T (1979) Medizinische Mykologie – ein praktischer Leitfaden. Editiones Roche, Basel Grenzach Wyhlen London

Wiedey KD, Kompa HE, Franz H (1984) Dosiswirkungs-Untersuchungen mit dem Polyenantimykotikum Natamycin in einem galenisch neu entwickelten Ovulum bei vaginalen Hefeinfektionen. Mykosen 27: 415

Winckel F (1866) Über die Bedeutung pflanzlicher Parasiten der Scheide bei Schwangeren. Berl klin Wschr 3: 237

Wise GJ, Goldberg Ph, Kozinn PhJ (1976) Genitourinary Candidiasis: Diagnosis and Treatment. J Urol 116: 788

Woodruff PW, Hesseltine HC (1938) Relationship of oral thrush to vaginal mycosis and the incidence of each. Am J Obstet Gynecol 30: 467

Wunderlich M (1979) Pilznachweis im Mammasekret. Mykosen 22: 115

Yarrow D, Meyer A (1978) Proposal for amendment of diagnosis of the genus Candida Berkhout nom cons. Intern J System Bacteriol 28 (4): 611

Ziegler HK, Veith G (1967) Hefeinfektionen im Neugeborenenalter. Arch Kinderheilk 175: 179

11 Pictures

11.1 Yeasts from A (albicans) to Z (zeylanoides)

Pure cultures and microscope slides* of facultatively pathogenic yeasts and some other important species.

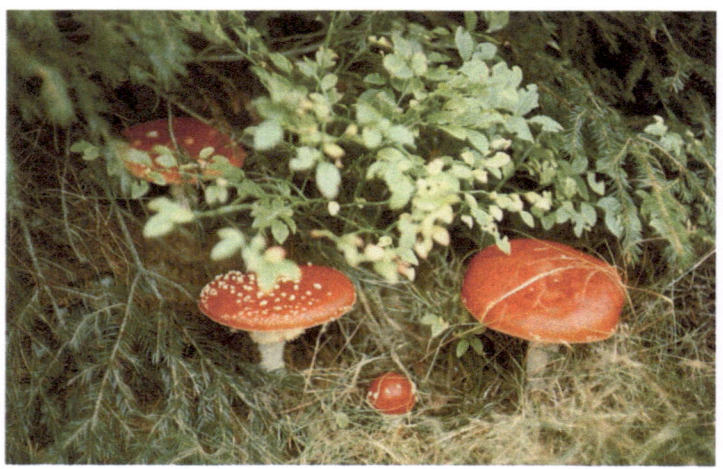

Fig. 1. Fly agaric *(Amanita muscaria)* – a handsome poisonous cap-forming fungus

---

* The pure cultures were kindly made available from the collections of the Mycological Laboratory of Bayer AG (Pharma-Forschungszentrum Wuppertal) or by Centraalbureau voor Schimmelcultures, Delft. Unless stated otherwise, all phase-contrast micrographs represent magnifications of × 400.

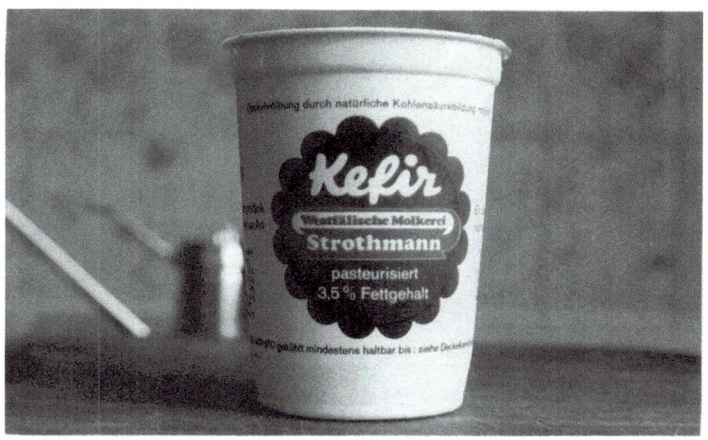

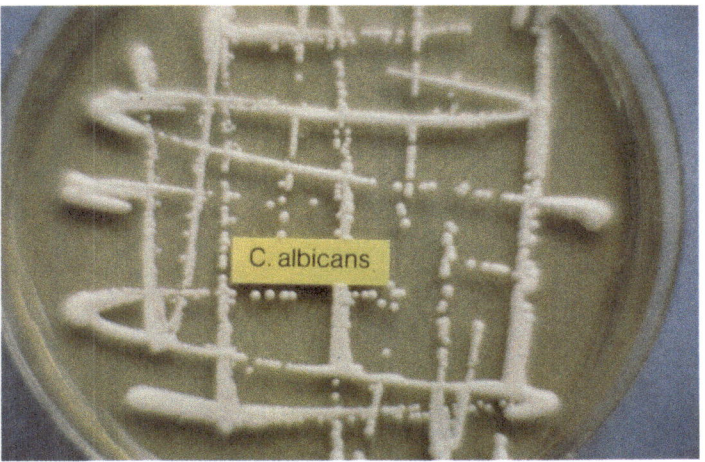

C. albicans

Fig. 2, 3. The spectrum of the 196 species of *Candida* ranges from the edible *Candida kefyr* to the sometimes fatal *Candida albicans*

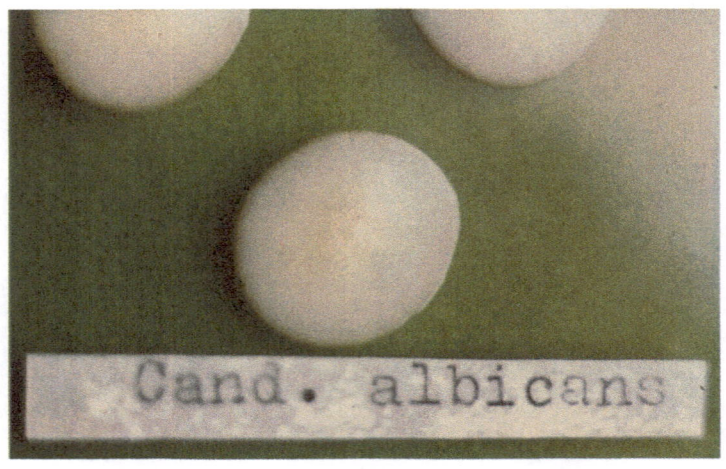

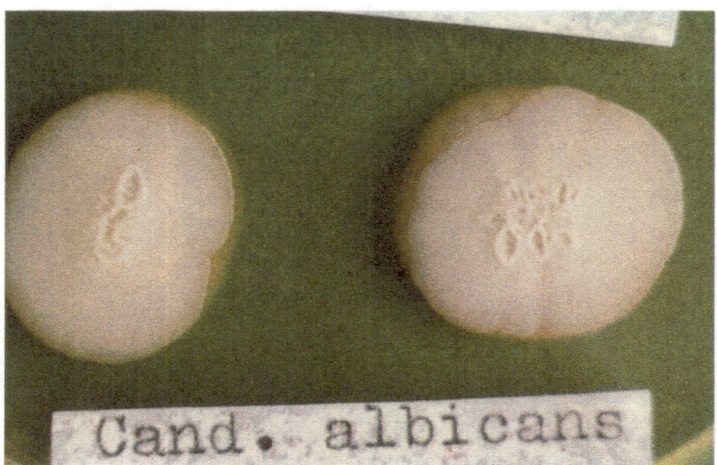

Fig. 4, 5. Pure cultures of two different strains of *Candida albicans* on Nervina agar according to Grütz-III

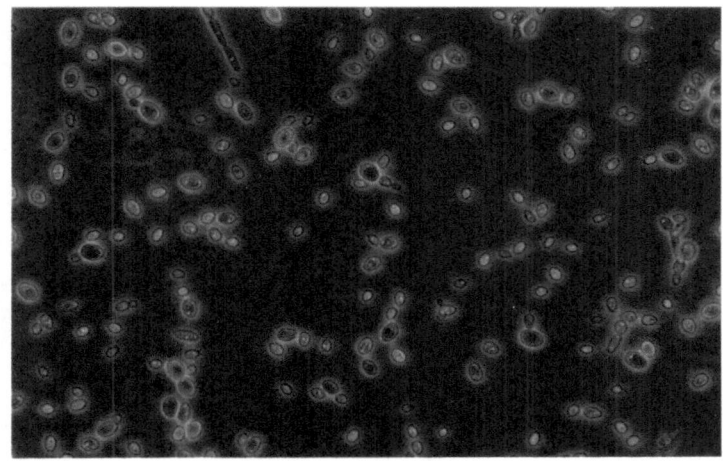

Fig. 6. *Candida albicans,* wet preparation from Nervina agar (Grütz III). Large oval blastospores and isolated pseudohyphae

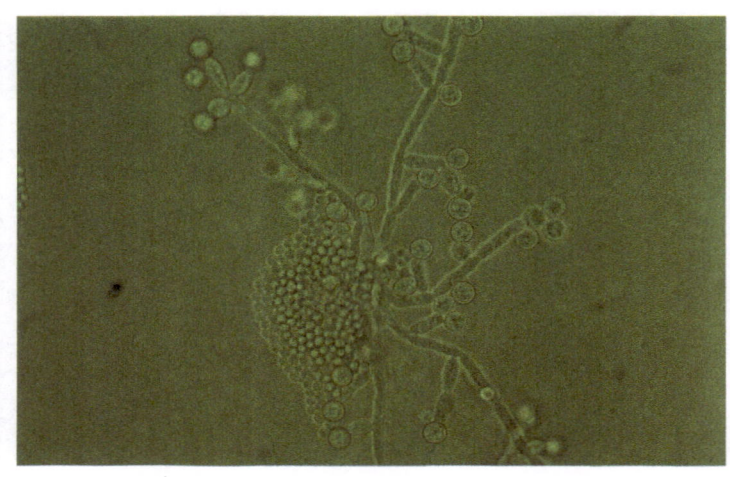

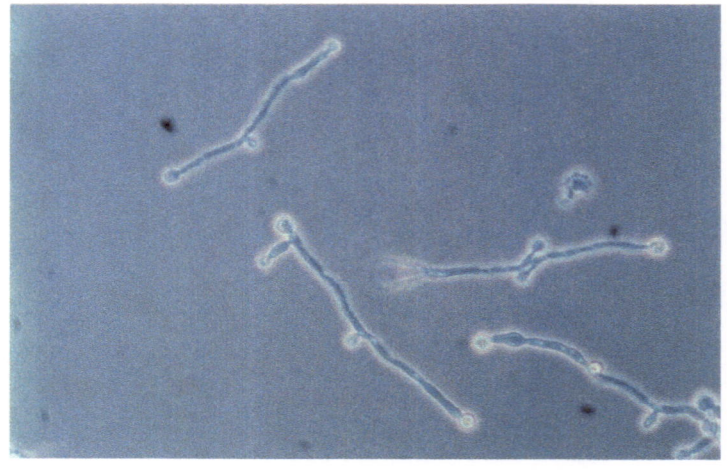

Fig. 7, 8. *Candida albicans* on rice agar. Blastospores, pseudohyphae and chlamydospores

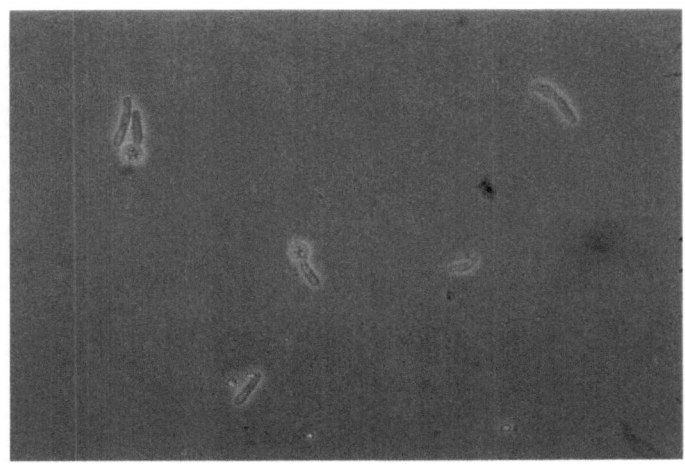

Fig. 9. *Candida albicans* after 4 hours in human serum. Formation of germ tubes

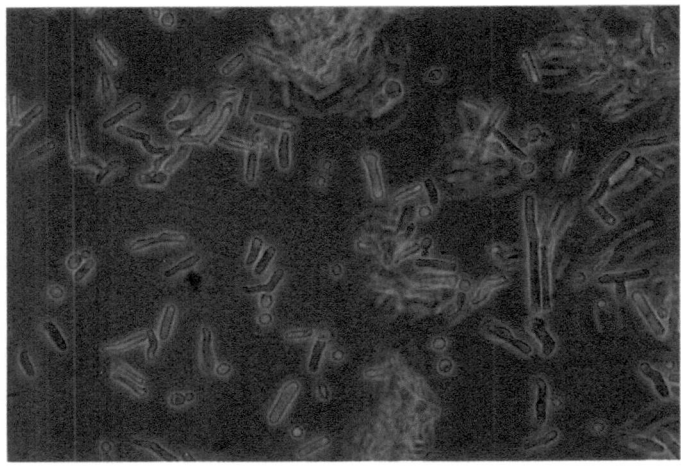

Fig. 10. *Candida albicans* after 24 hours in human serum. Germ tubes

73

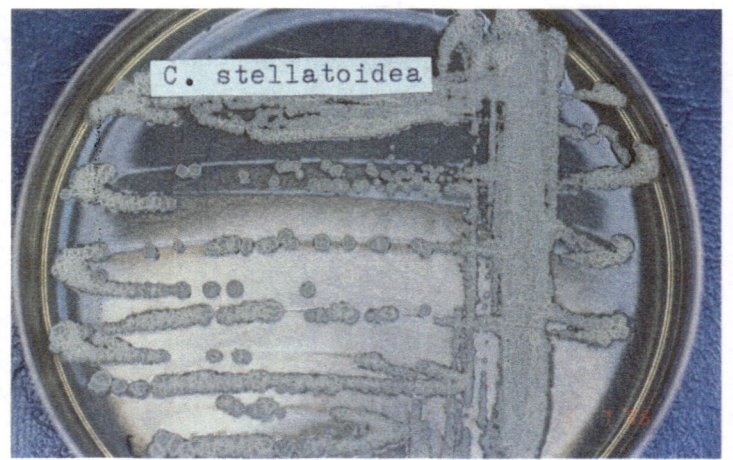

Fig. 11. *Candida stellatoidea (syn. albicans)* on Sabouraud's 2% glucose agar

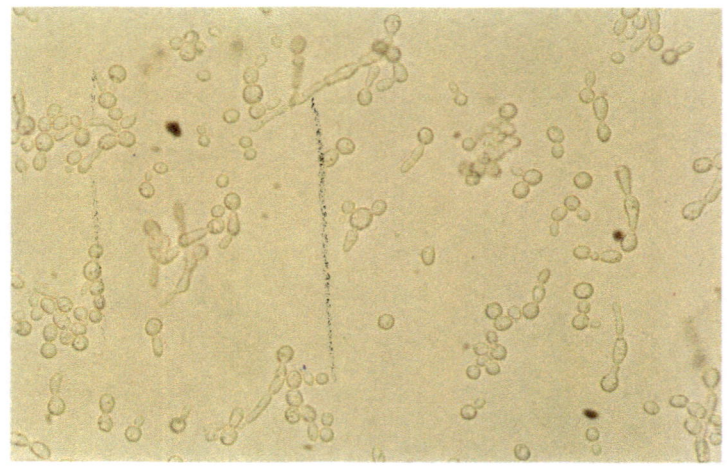

Fig. 12. *Candida stellatoidea* (syn. *albicans*). Wet preparation from Nervina agar according to Grütz III (bright ground microscopy)

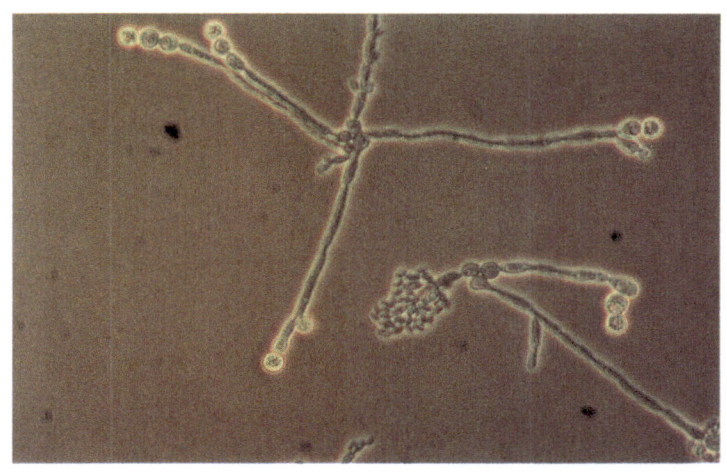

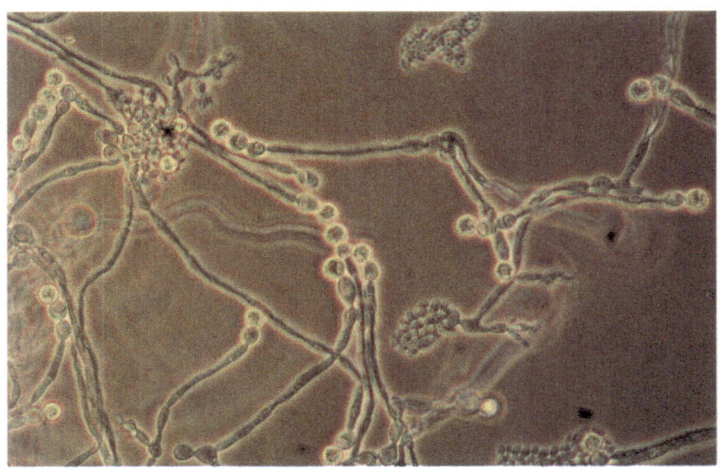

Fig. 13, 14. *Candida stellatoidea* (syn. *albicans*) on rice agar after 48 hours. Chlamydospores and protochlamydospores on the pseudohyphae

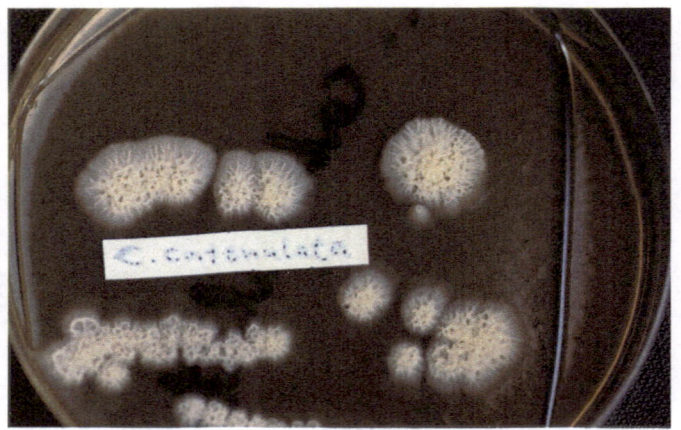

Fig. 15. *Candida catenulata (brumptii)* on Nervina (Grütz III)

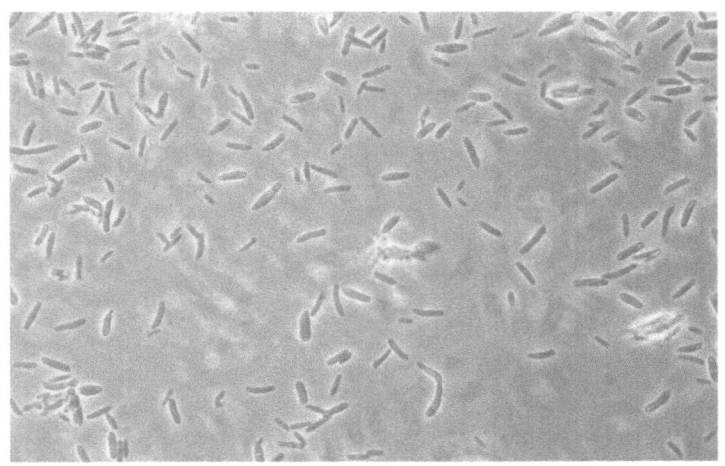

Fig. 16. *Candida catenulata (brumptii).* Wet preparation from Nervina agar (Grütz III). Large, oblong budding cells, isolated pseudohyphae

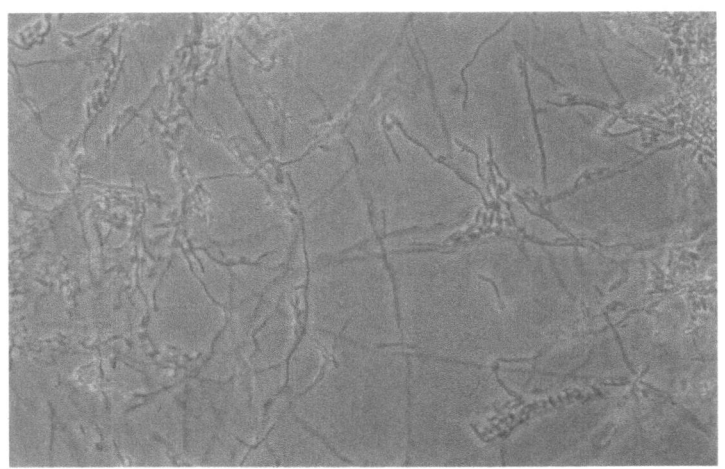

Fig. 17. *Candida catenulata (brumptii)* on rice agar (20 hours), Long, thin pseudomycelium

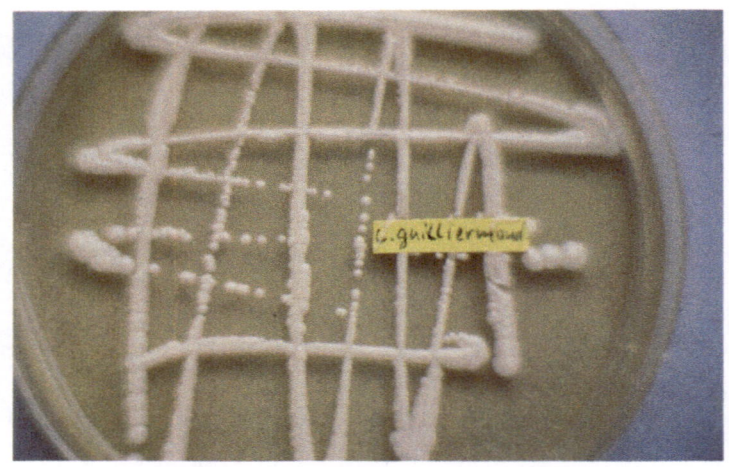

Fig. 18. *Candida guilliermondii* on Sabouraud's 2% glucose agar

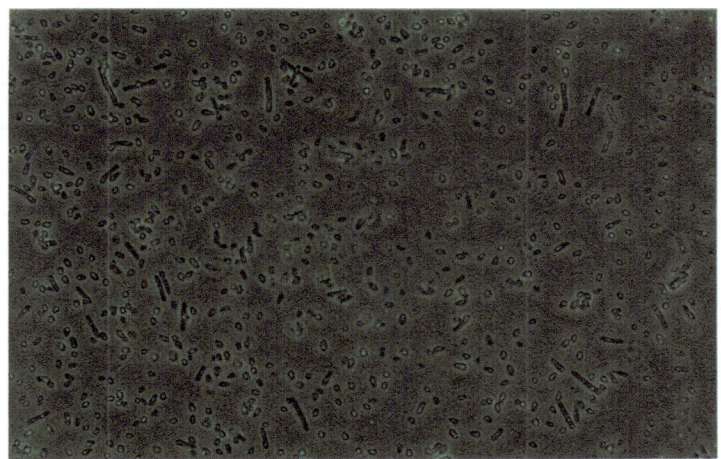

Fig. 19. *Candida guilliermondii* in a wet preparation from Nervina agar (Grütz III)

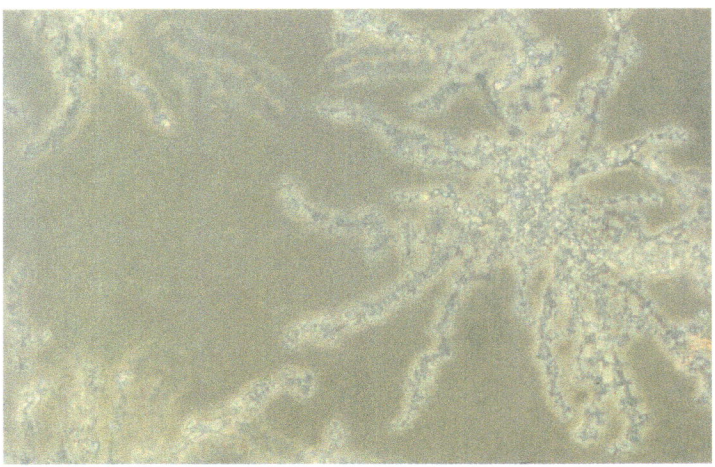

Fig. 20. *Candida guilliermondii* on rice agar (48 hours). Small, roundish to oval budding cells and thin branching pseudomycelium. Some strains do not form pseudohyphae and because of similar metabolic characteristics, are even biochemically difficult to distinguish from *Candida famata*

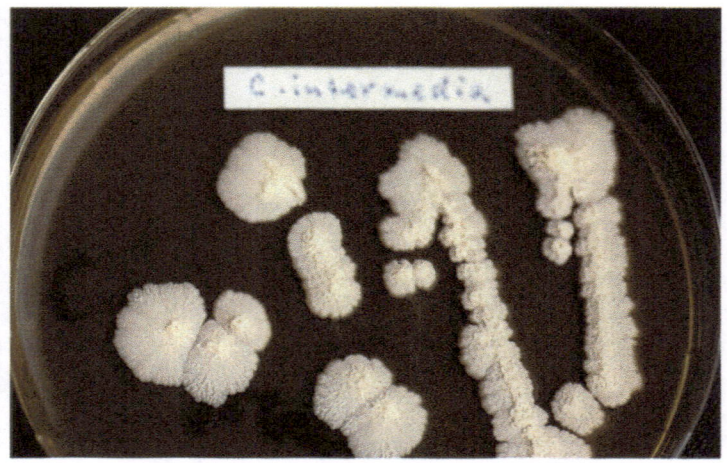

Fig. 21. *Candida intermedia* on Nervina agar (Grütz III)

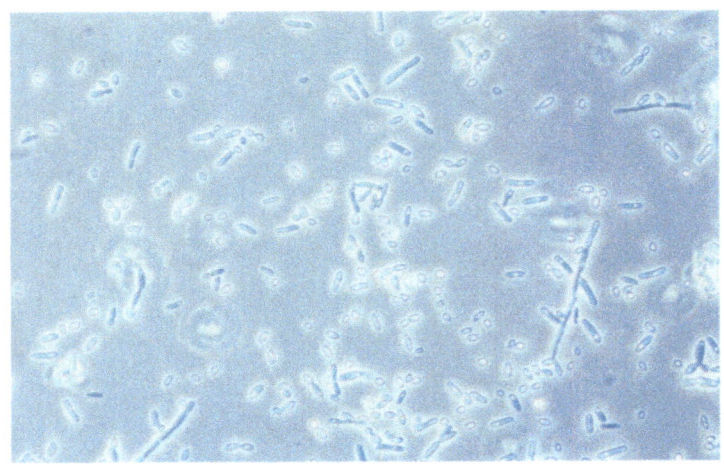

Fig. 22. *Candida intermedia* in a wet preparation from Nervina agar (Grütz III)

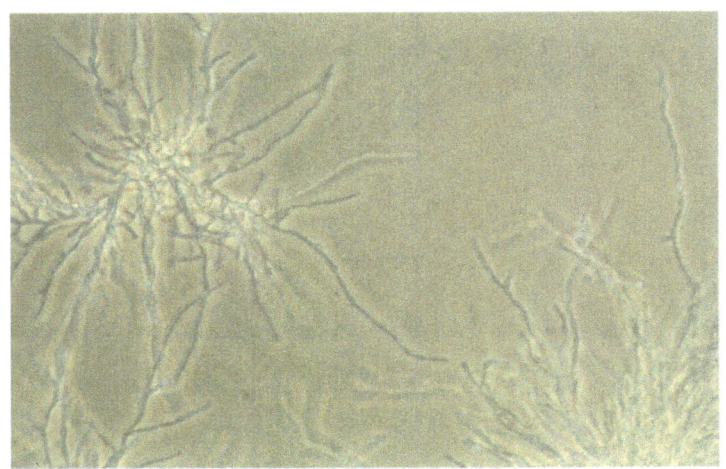

Fig. 23. *Candida intermedia* on rice agar (26 hours). Branched pseudomycelia

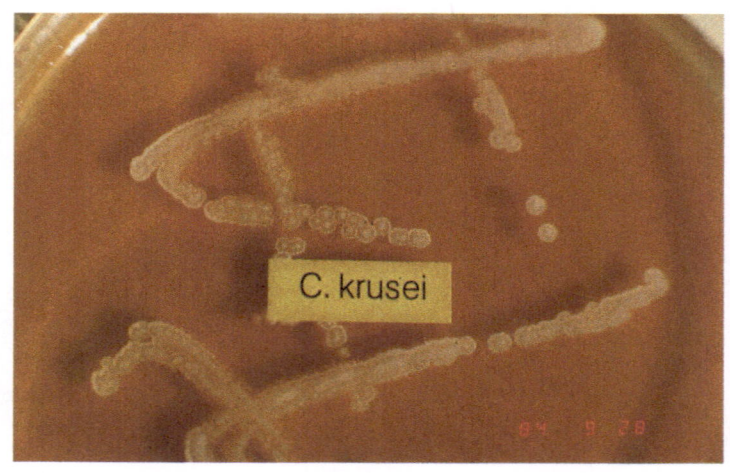

C. krusei

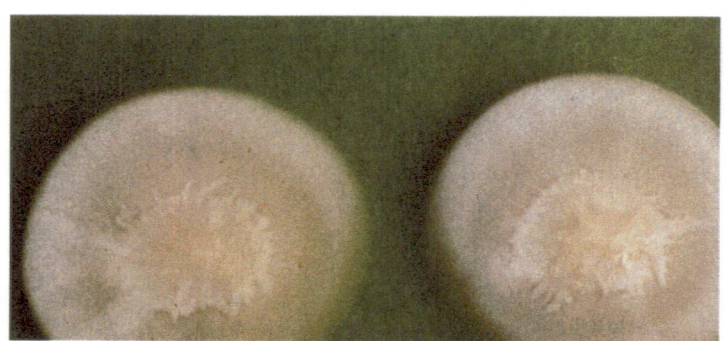

Fig. 24, 25. *Candida krusei* on Nervina agar (Grütz III)

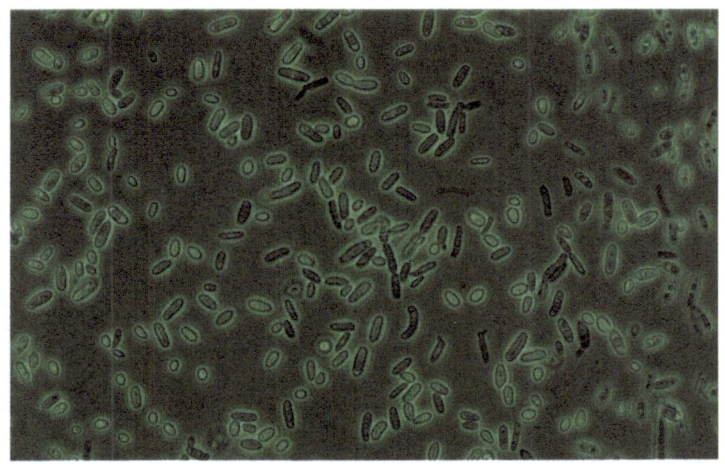

Fig. 26. *Candida krusei* in a wet preparation from Nervina agar (Grütz III)

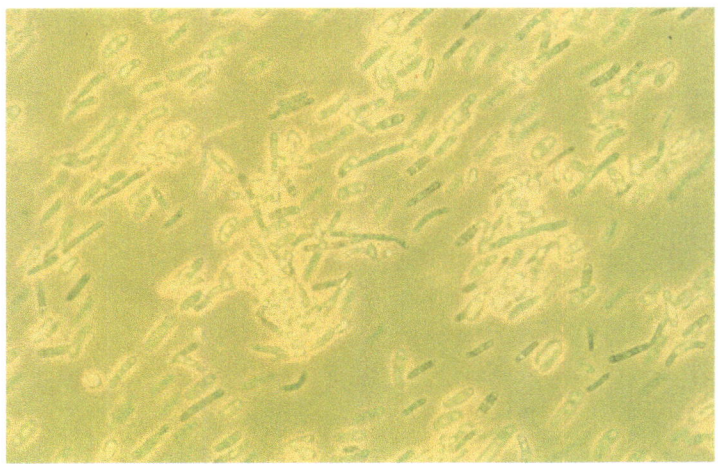

Fig. 27. *Candida krusei*. Wet preparation from a 10-week old Nervina agar plate (Grütz III). Typical elongated large budding cells, often dark, vacuoles

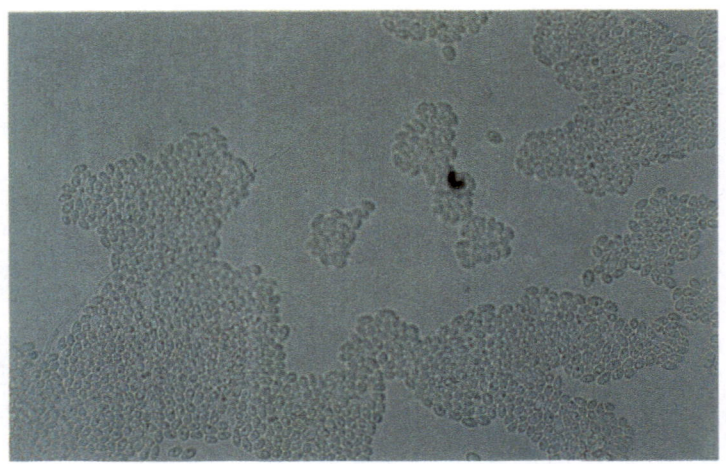

Fig. 28. *Candida krusei* on rice agar, here without formation of pseudohyphae. The thin mycelium is a mold contaminant

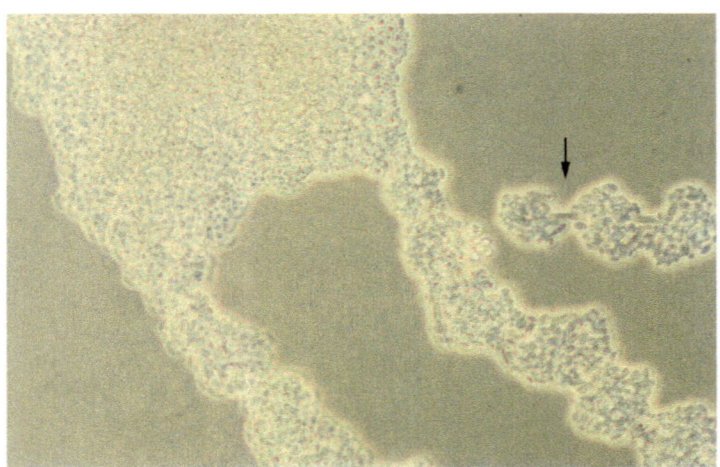

Fig. 29. *Candida krusei* on rice agar. Not every strain forms a pseudomycelium which in this case is rendered almost invisible by surrounding budding cells **(arrow)**

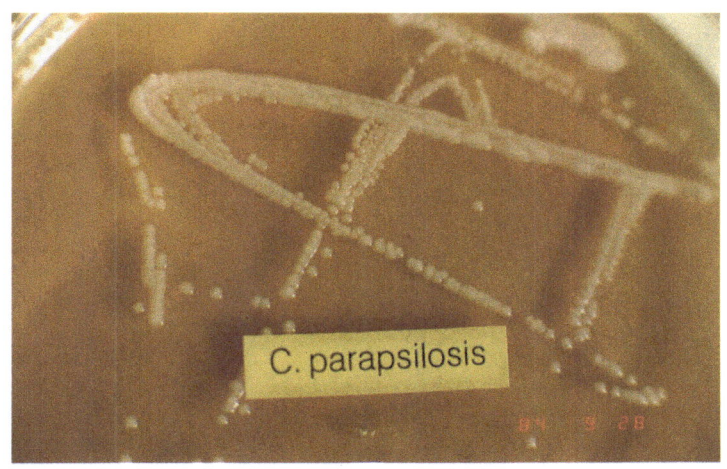

Fig. 30. *Candida parapsilosis* on Sabouraud's 2% glucose agar

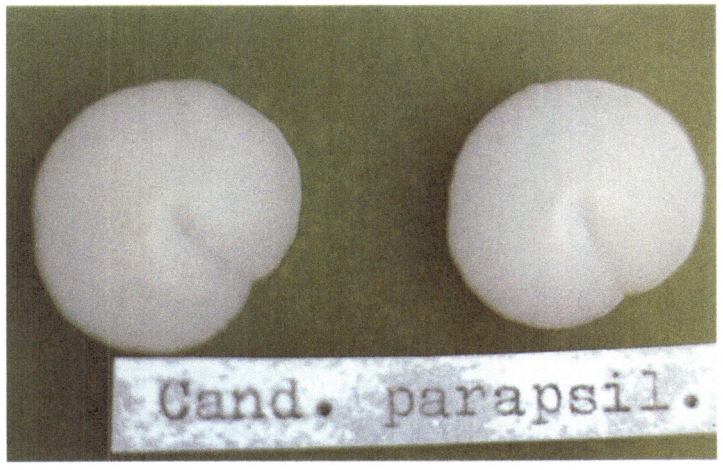

Fig. 31. *Candida parapsilosis* on Nervina agar (Grütz III)

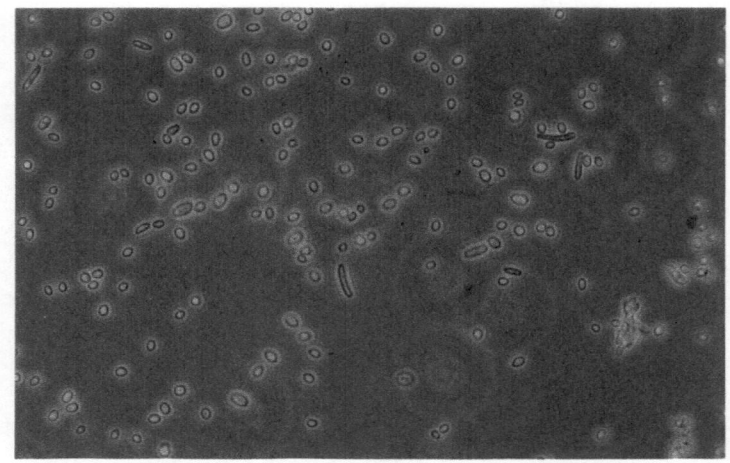

Fig. 32. *Candida parapsilosis* in a wet preparation from Nervina agar (Grütz III)

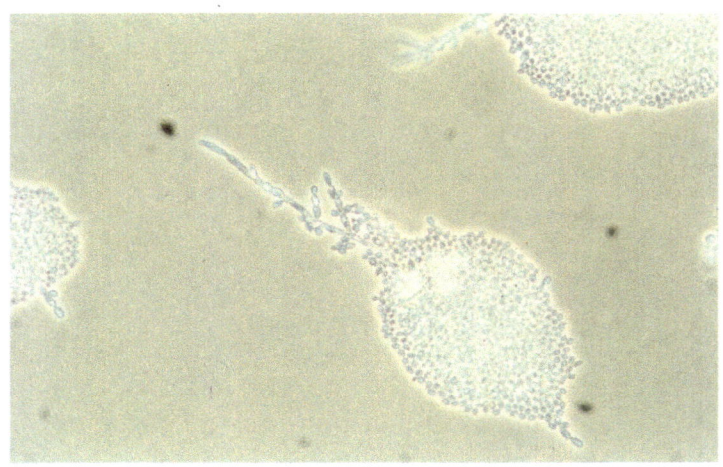

Fig. 33. *Candida parapsilosis* on rice agar (48 hours)

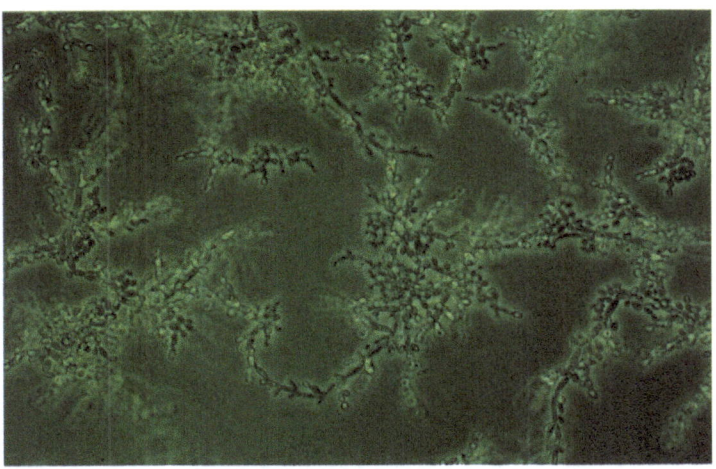

Fig. 34. *Candida parapsilosis* on rice agar (48 hours). Pseudomycelium with small round budding cells

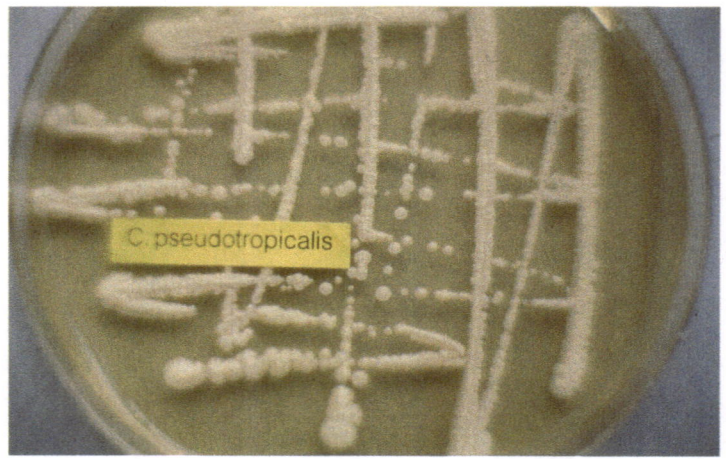

Fig. 35. *Candida kefyr (pseudotropicalis)* on Sabouraud's 2% glucose agar

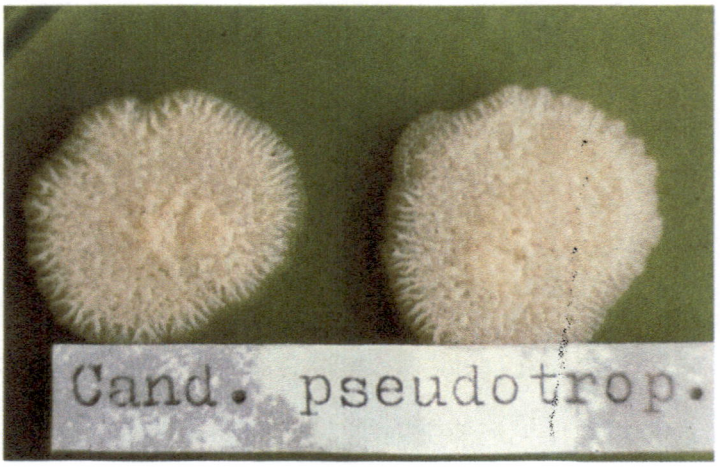

Fig. 36. *Candida kefyr (pseudotropicalis)* on Nervina agar (Grütz III)

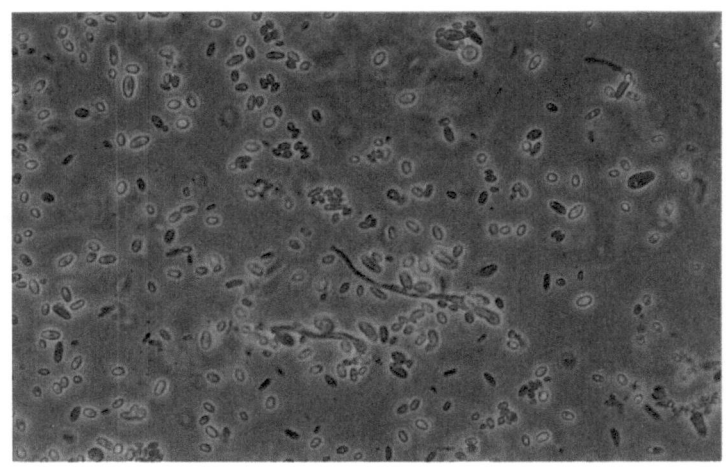

Fig. 37. *Candida kefyr (pseudotropicalis).* Wet preparation from Nervina agar (Grütz III)

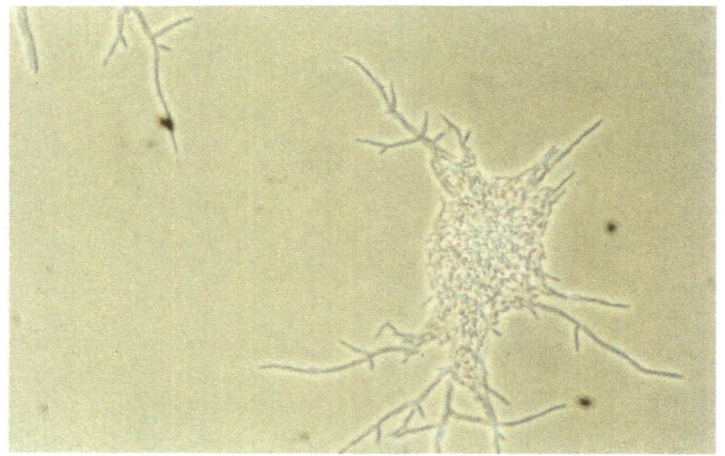

Fig. 38. *Candida kefyr (pseudotropicalis)* on rice agar (48 hours). Budding cells and thin branching pseudohyphae

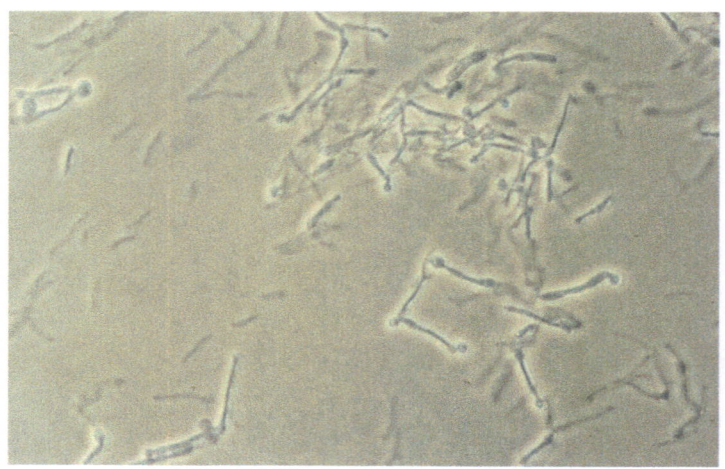

Fig. 39. *Candida kefyr (pseudotropicalis)* on rice agar (48 hours). Thin branching pseudohyphae and budding cells resembling chlamydospores

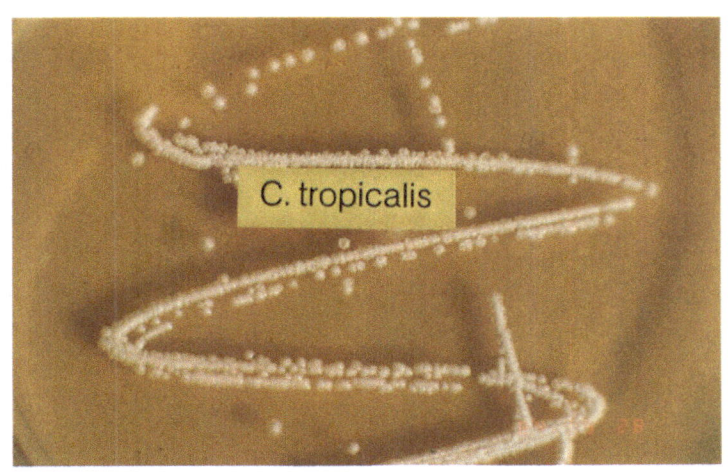

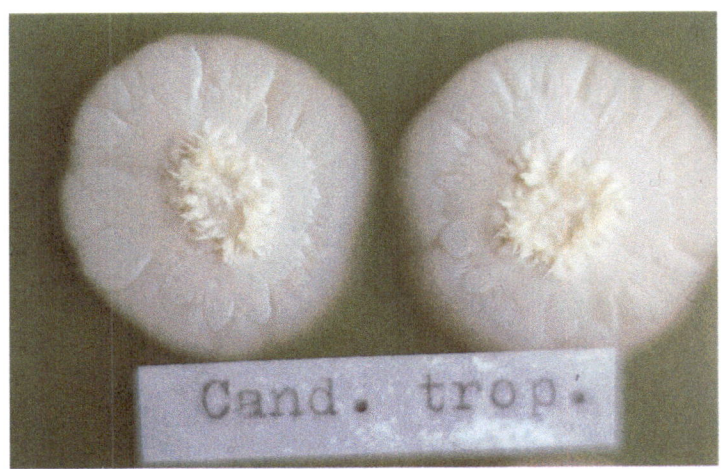

Fig. 40, 41. *Candida tropicalis* on Nervina agar (Grütz-III)

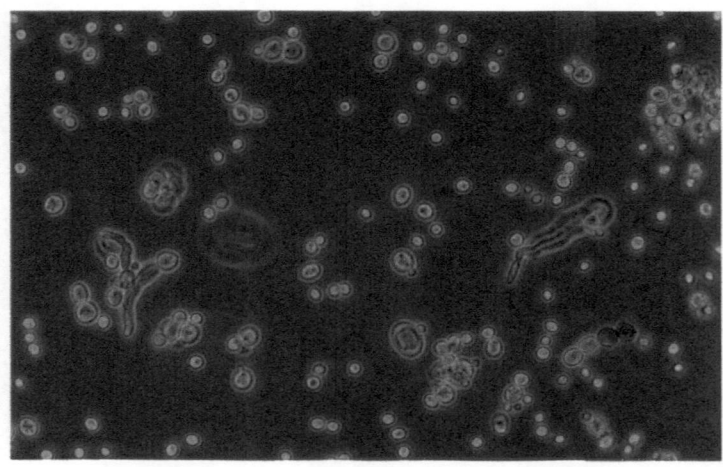

Fig. 42. *Candida tropicalis*. Wet preparation from a pure culture

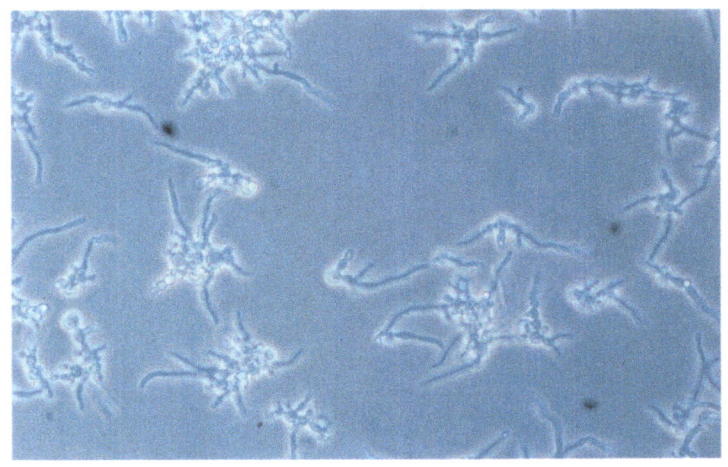

Fig. 43. *Candida tropicalis* on rice agar (20 h)

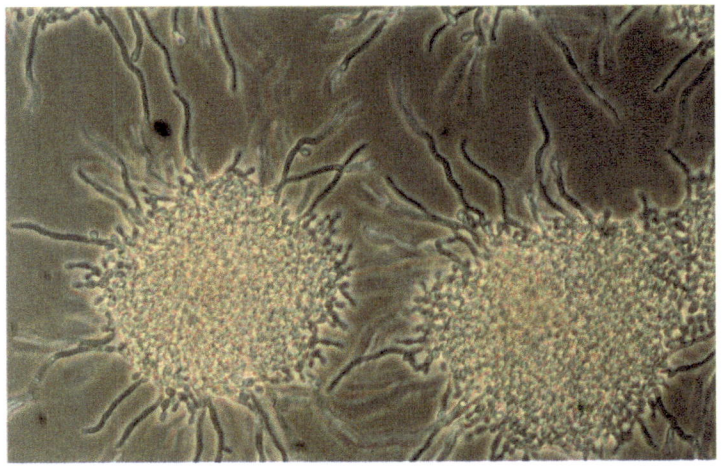

Fig. 44. *Candida tropicalis* on rice agar (48 h)

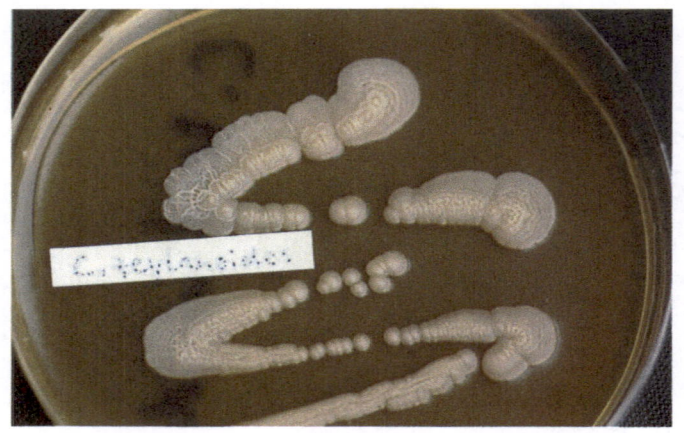

Fig. 45. *Candida zeylanoides* on Nervina agar (Grütz-III)

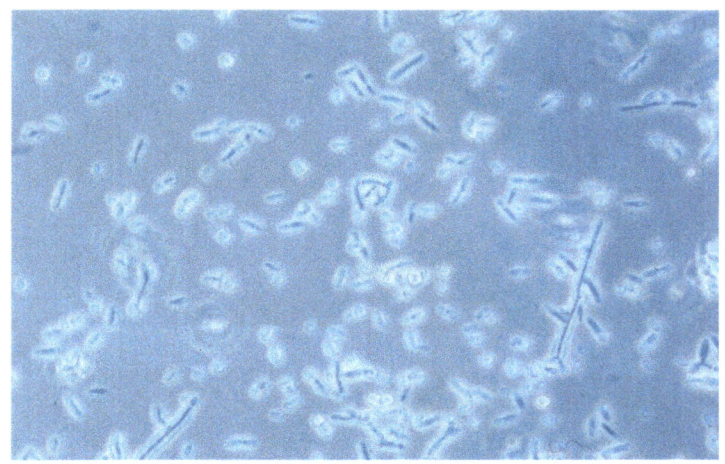

Fig. 46. *Candida zeylanoides* in a wet preparation from Nervina agar (Grütz-III)

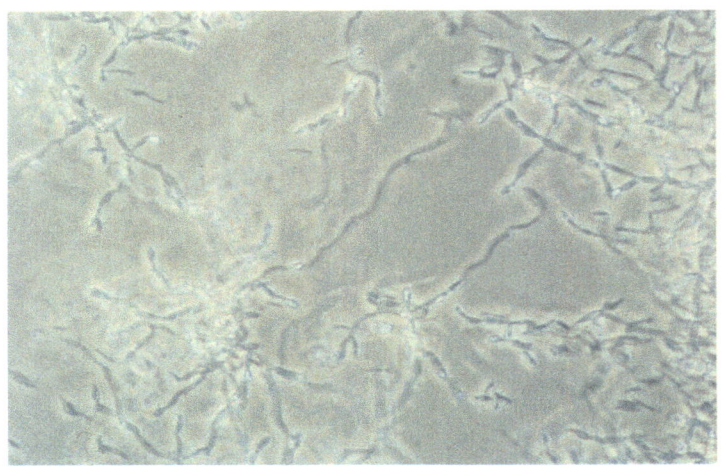

Fig. 47. *Candida zeylanoides* on rice agar (26 h). Thin pseudohyphae

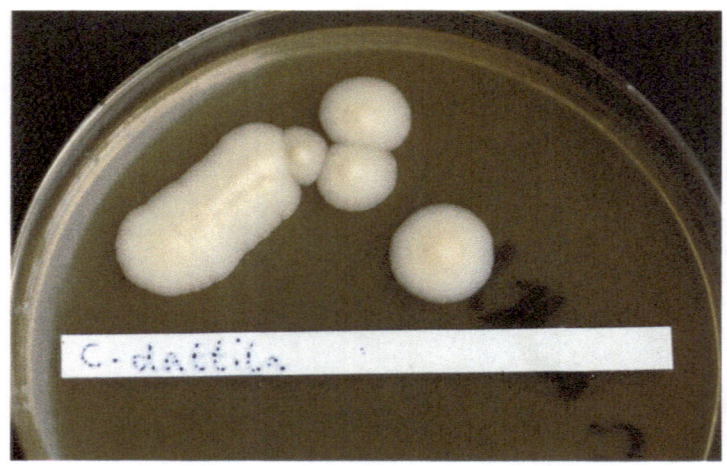

Fig. 48. *Candida dattila (Torulopsis dattila)* on Nervina agar (Grütz III)

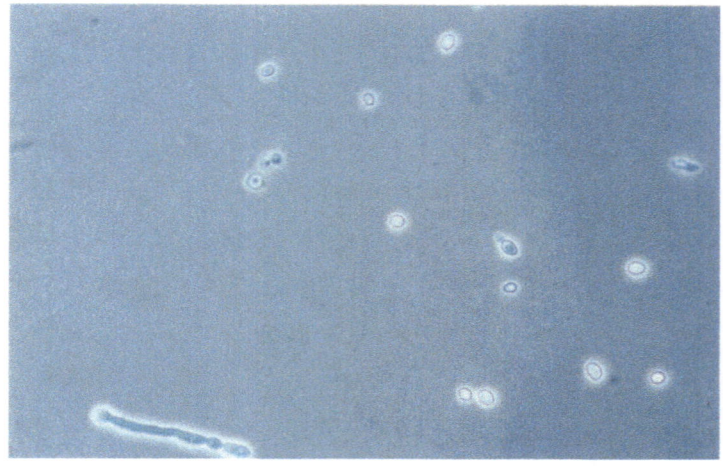

Fig. 49. *Candida dattila (Torulopsis dattila)* in a wet preparation from Nervina agar (Grütz III)

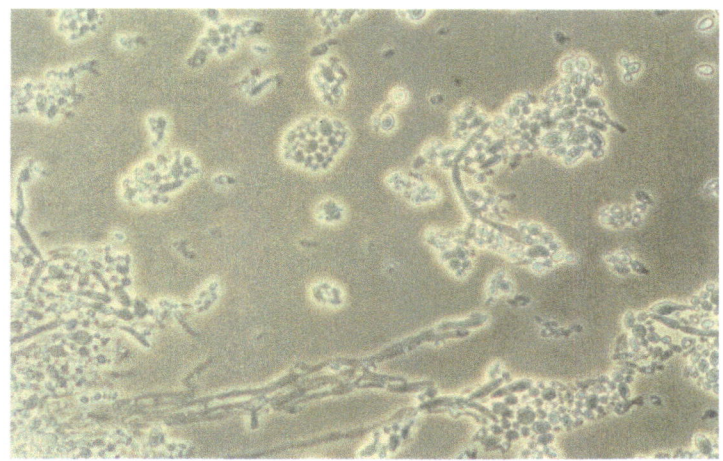

Fig. 50. *Candida dattila (Torulopsis dattila)* on rice agar (48 h). Budding cells, a few grossly bloated, with formation of pseudohyphae

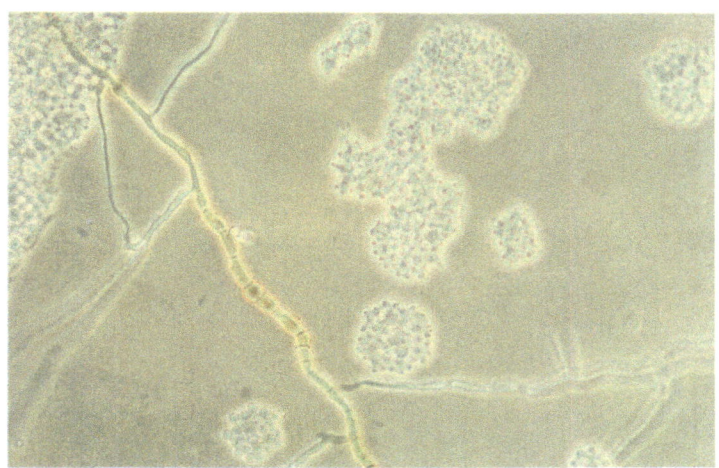

Fig. 51. *Candida dattila (Torulopsis dattila)* on rice agar. Budding cells only; the septate, branching mycelium emanates from a mold

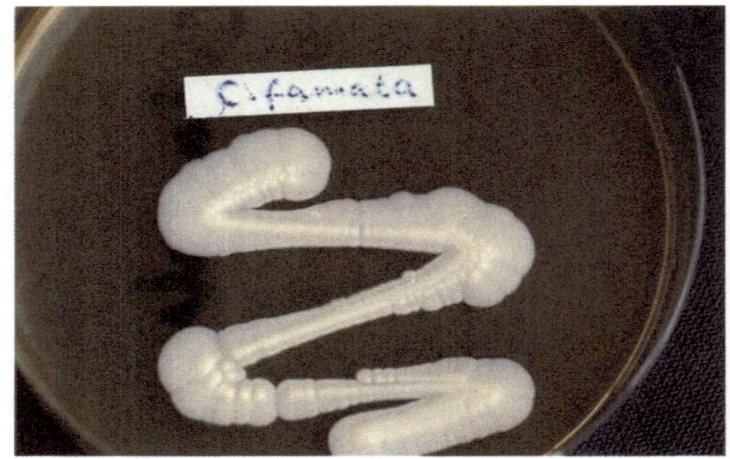

Fig. 52. *Candida famata (Torulopsis candida)* on Nervina agar (Grütz-III)

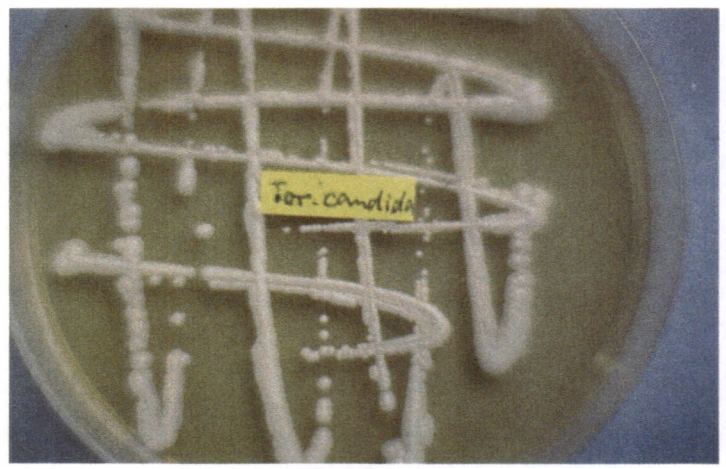

Fig. 53. *Candida famata (Torulopsis candida)* on Sabouraud's 2% glucose agar

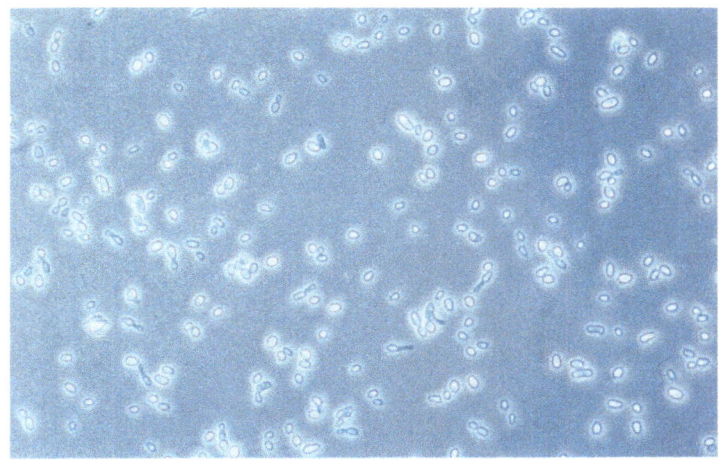

Fig. 54. *Candida famata (Torulopsis candida),* wet preparation from Nervina agar (Grütz-III). Budding cells and short pseudohyphae

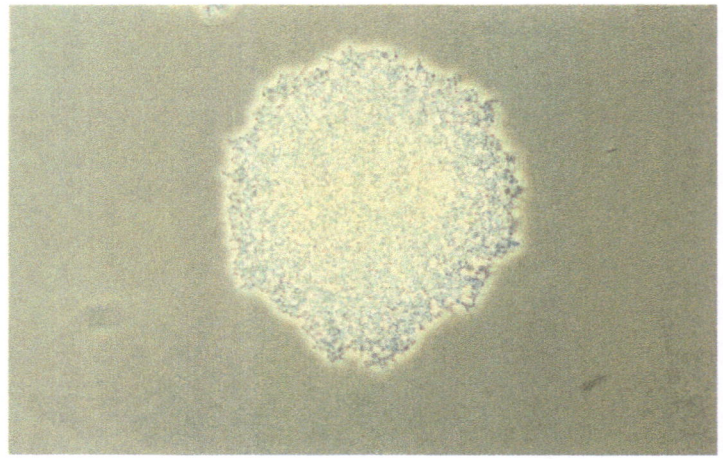

Fig. 55. *Candida famata (Torulopsis candida)* on rice agar (48 h). Very small roundish-to oval budding cells without pseudohyphae

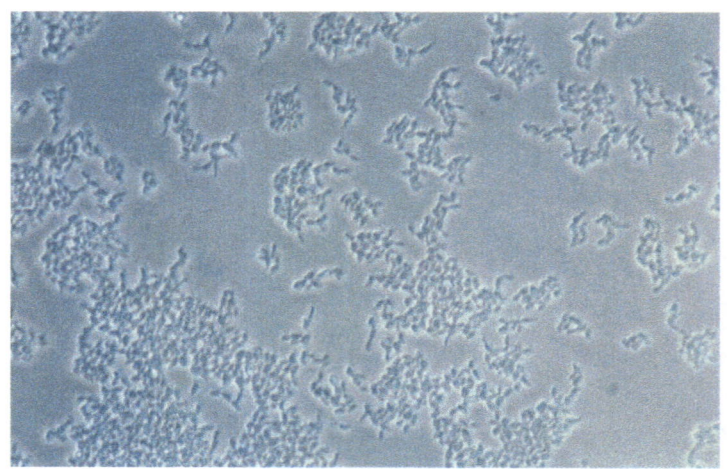

Fig. 56. *Candida famata (Torulopsis candida)* on rice agar (24 h). Budding cells and rudimentary pseudohyphae

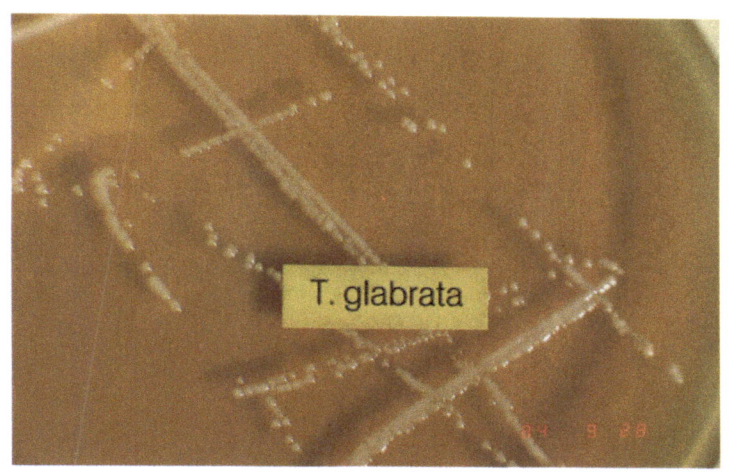

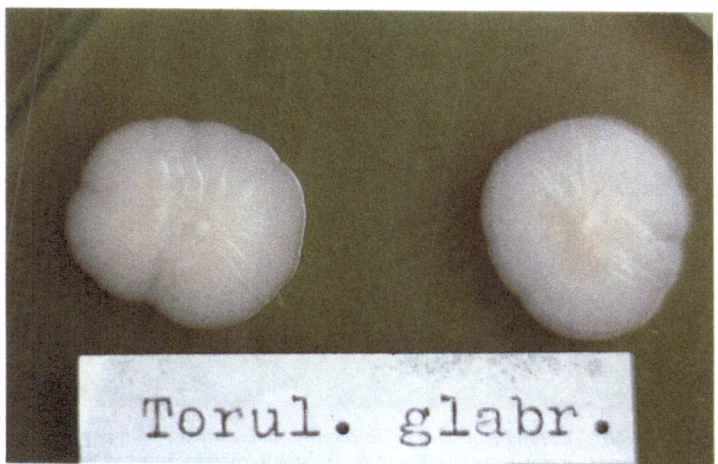

Fig. 57, 58. *Candida glabrata (Torulopsis glabrata)* on Nervina agar (Grütz-III)

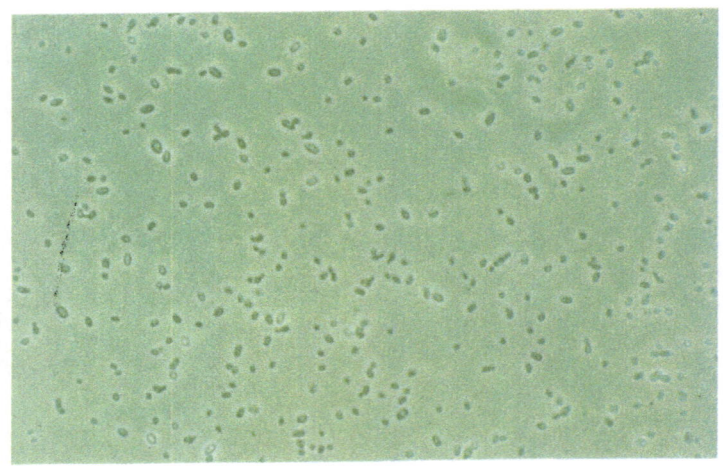

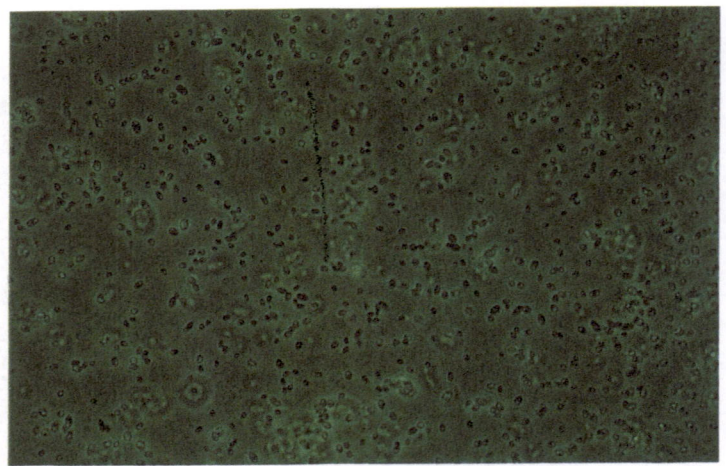

Fig. 59, 60. *Candida glabrata (Torulopsis glabrata)* in a wet preparation from Nervina agar (Grütz III). Relatively small, oval budding cells often appearing dark

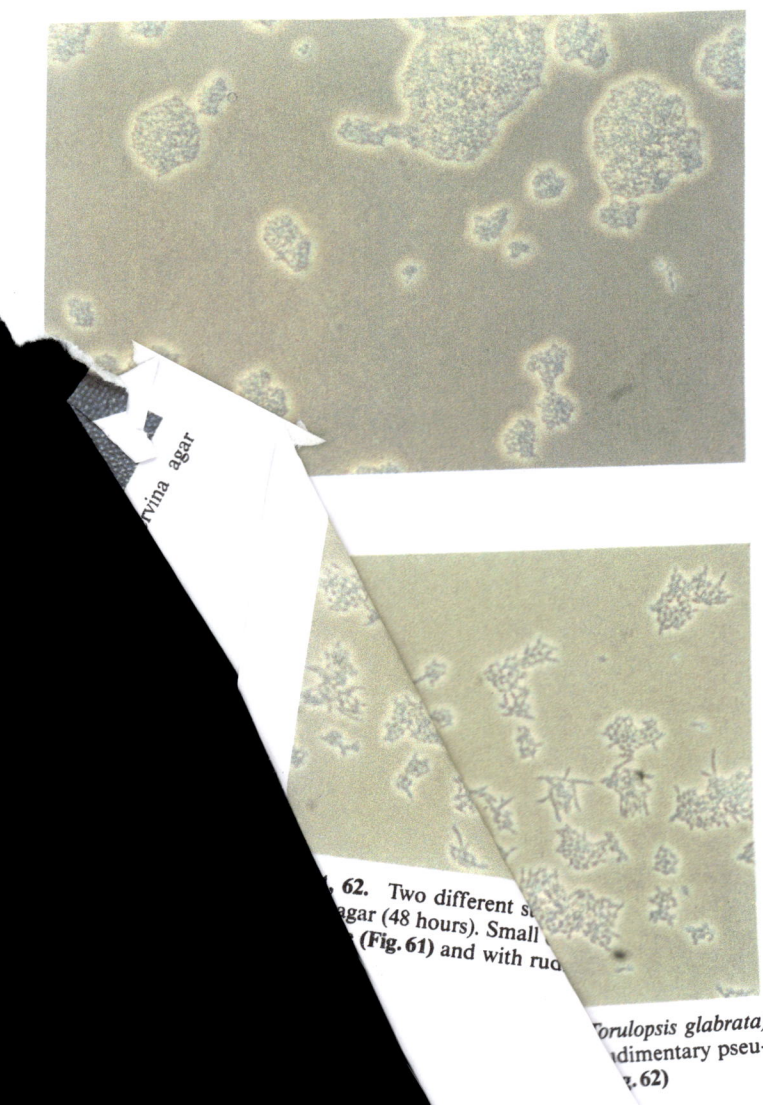

rvina agar

62. Two different s
agar (48 hours). Small
s **(Fig. 61)** and with rud

Torulopsis glabrata)
dimentary pseu-
g. 62)

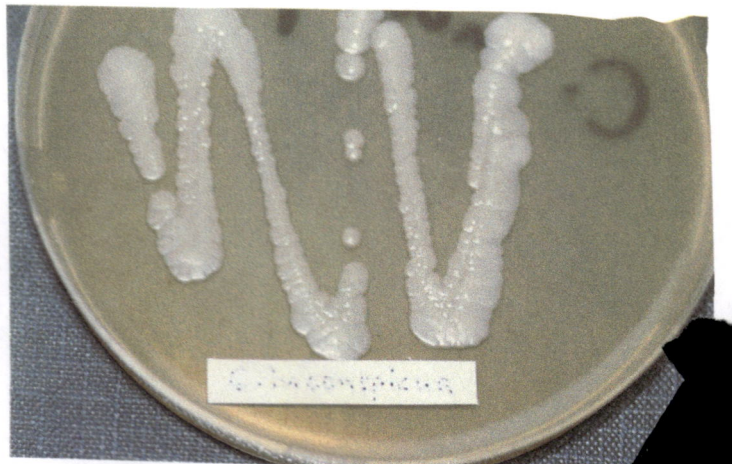

Fig. 63. *Candida inconspicua (Torulopsis inconspicua)* on N
(Grütz-III)

Fig. 6
on rice
dohypha

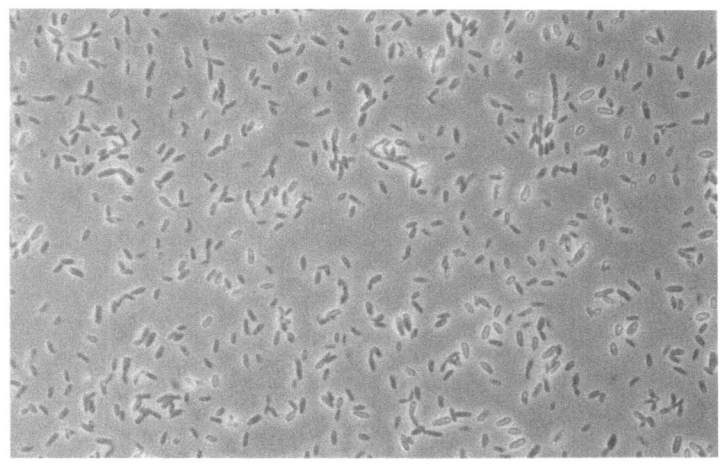

Fig. 64. *Candida inconspicua (Torulopsis inconspicua)* in a wet preparation from Nervina agar (Grütz-III)

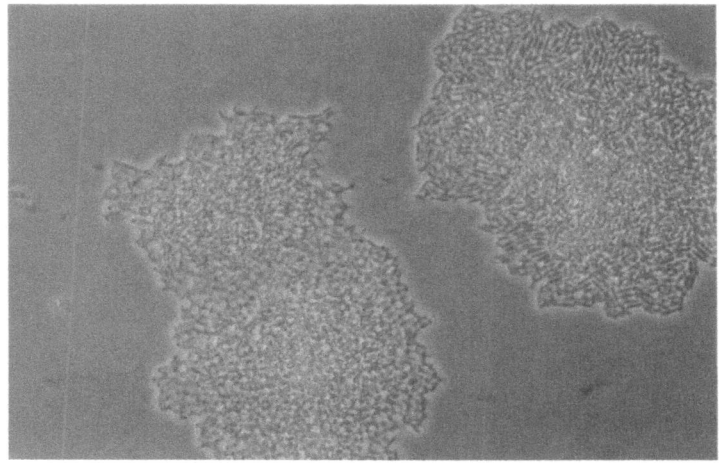

Fig. 65. *Candida inconspicua (Torulopsis inconspicua)* on rice agar (26 h). Budding cells and short pseudohyphae

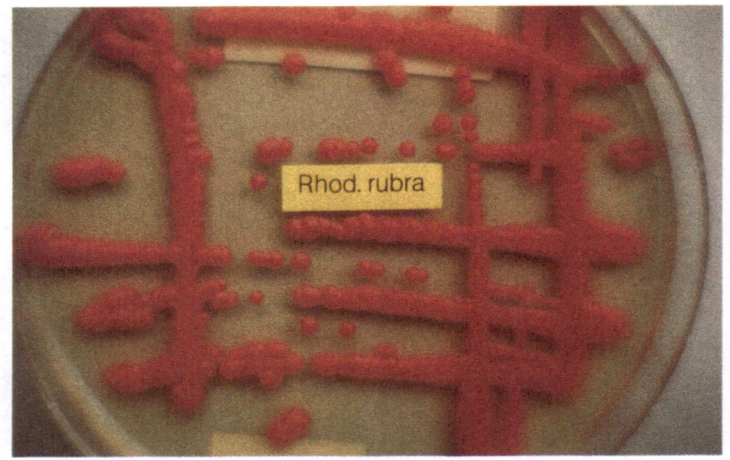

Fig. 66. *Rhodotorula rubra* on Sabouraud's 2% glucose agar

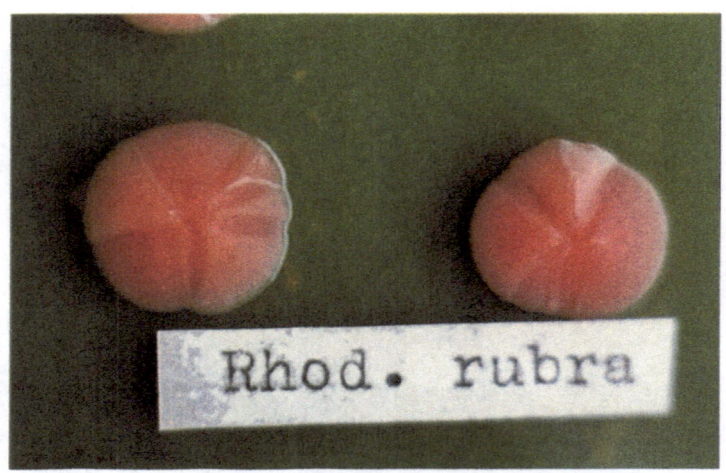

Fig. 67. *Rhodotorula rubra* on Nervina agar (Grütz-III)

106

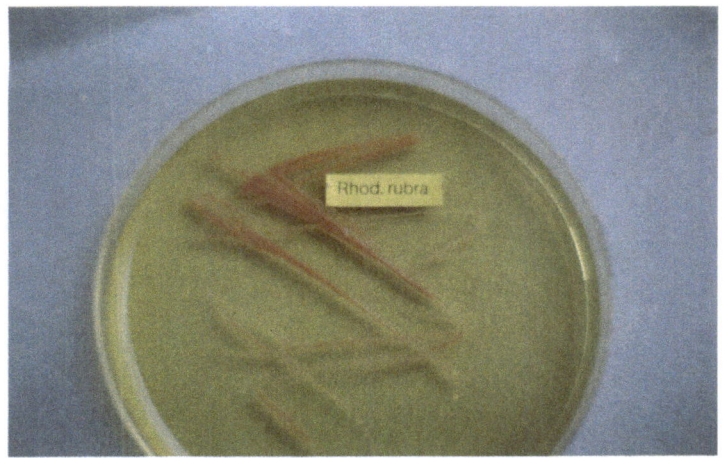

Fig. 68. *Rhodotorula rubra* on Candida II agar

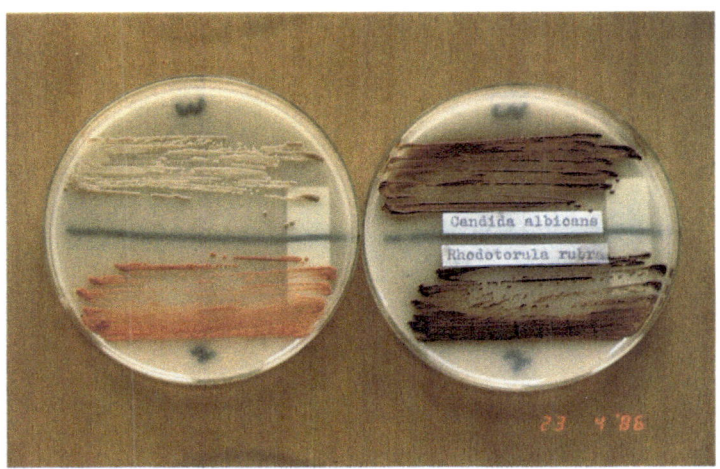

Fig. 69. *Rhodotorula rubra* on two different Nickersons' agar plates together with *Candida albicans*

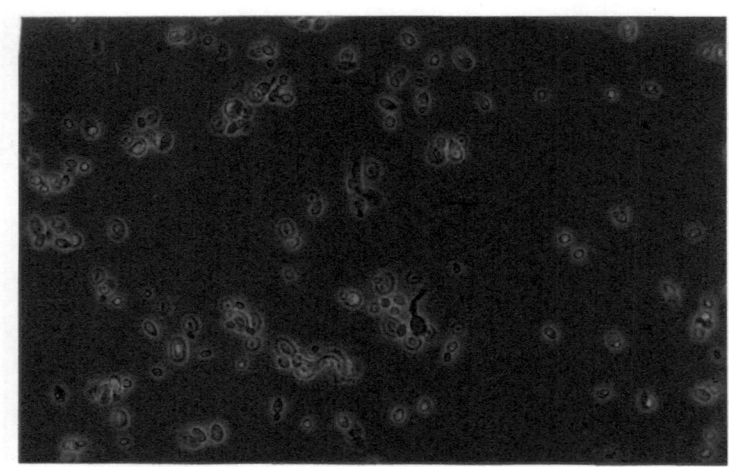

Fig. 70. *Rhodotorula rubra* in a wet preparation

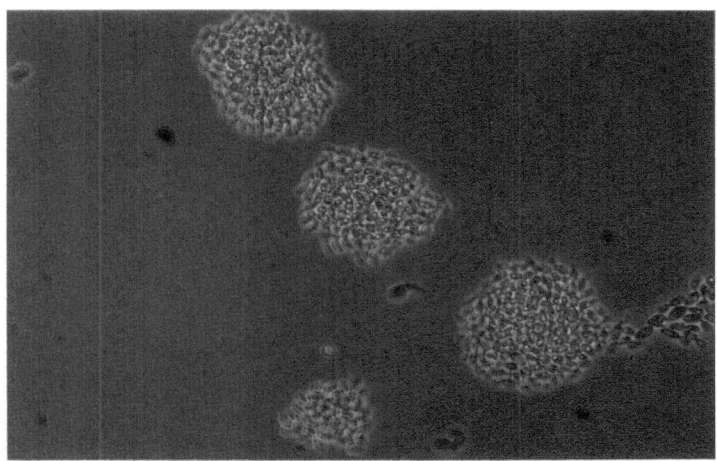

Fig. 71. *Rhodotorula rubra* on rice agar (48 h). Budding cells with light nuclei, no pseudohyphae

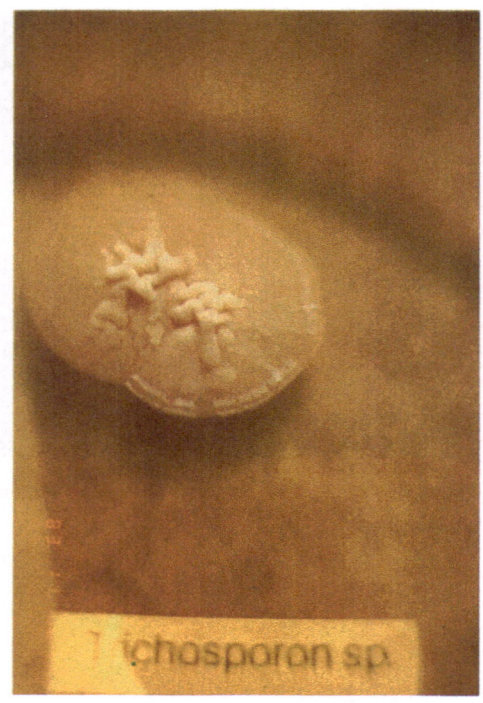

Fig. 72. *Trichosporon cutaneum (beigelii)* on Nervina agar (Grütz-III)

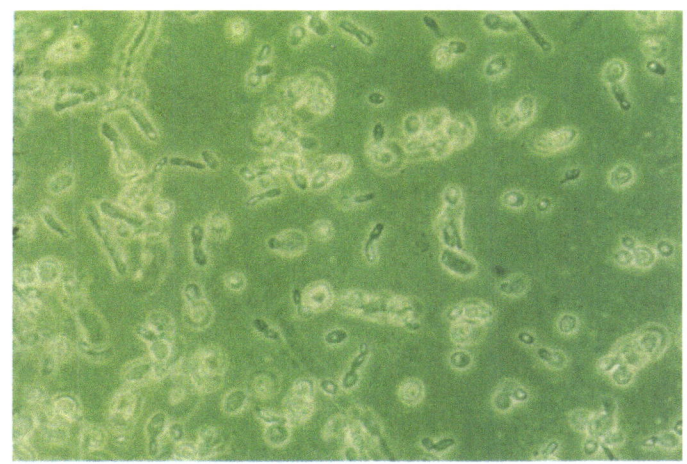

Fig. 73. *Trichosporon cutaneum (beigelii).* Blastospores and mycelia (not clearly discernible here)

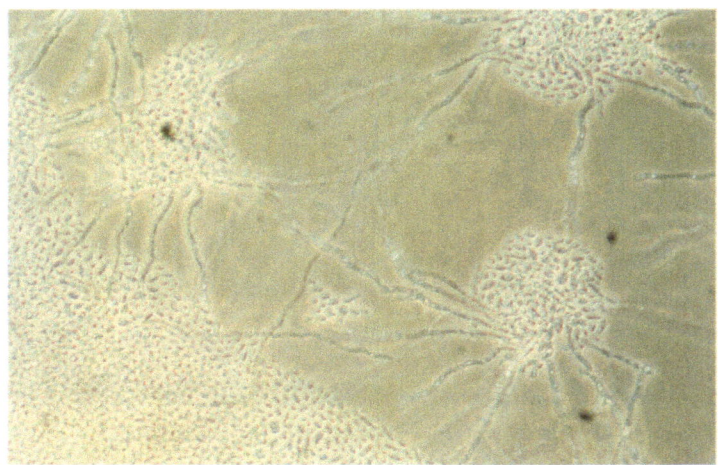

Fig. 74. *Trichosporon cutaneum (beigelii)* on rice agar (48 h). Mycelium, budding cells and isolated arthrospores

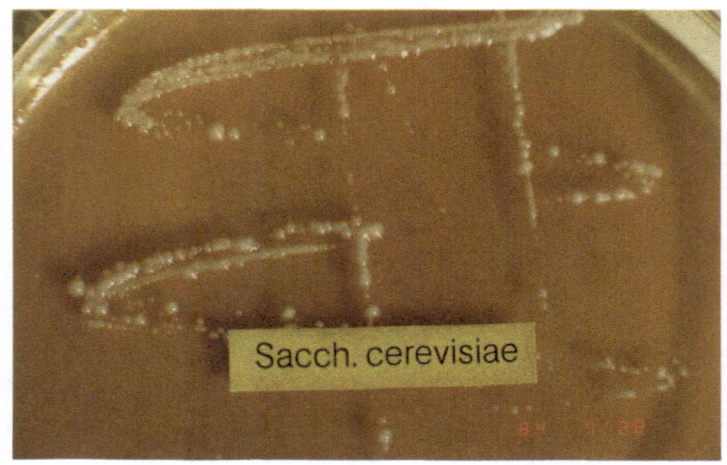

Sacch. cerevisiae

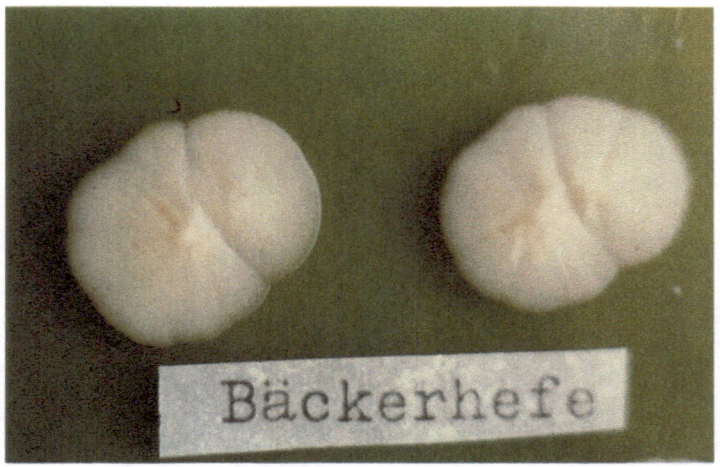

Bäckerhefe

Fig. 75, 76. *Saccharomyces cerevisiae* on Nervina agar (Grütz-III)

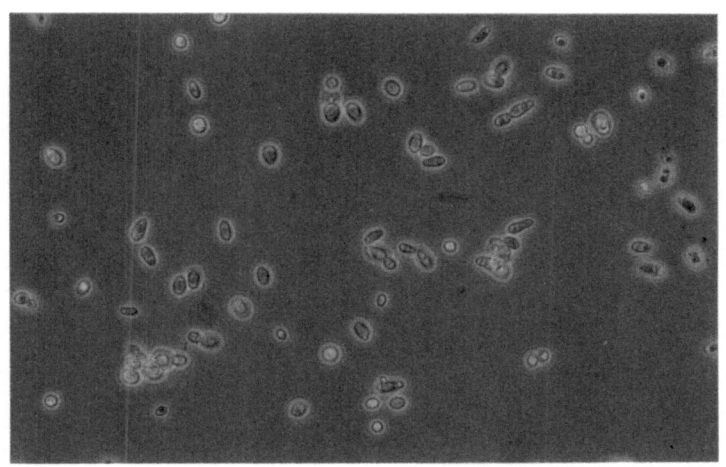

Fig. 77. *Saccharomyces cerevisiae* in a wet preparation from Nervina agar (Grütz-III)

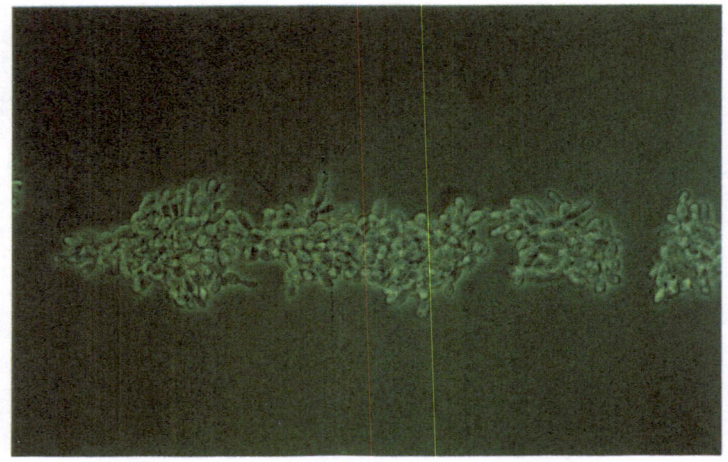

Fig. 78. *Saccharomyces cerevisiae* on rice agar. Blastospores and rudimentary pseudohyphae

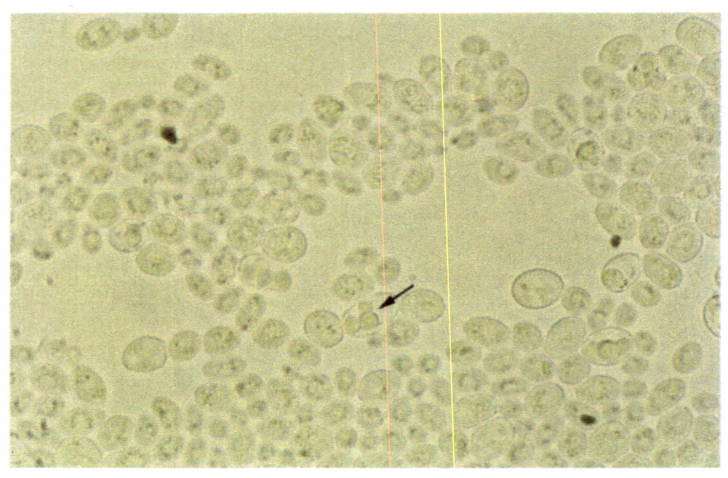

Fig. 79. *Saccharomyces cerevisiae* on rice agar (48 h) (magnification ×1000). Budding cells and ascospores **(arrow)**

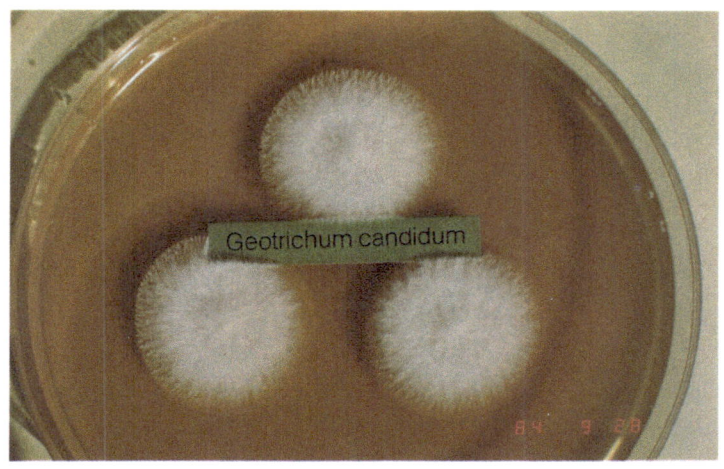

Fig. 80. *Geotrichum candidum* on Nervina agar (Grütz-III)

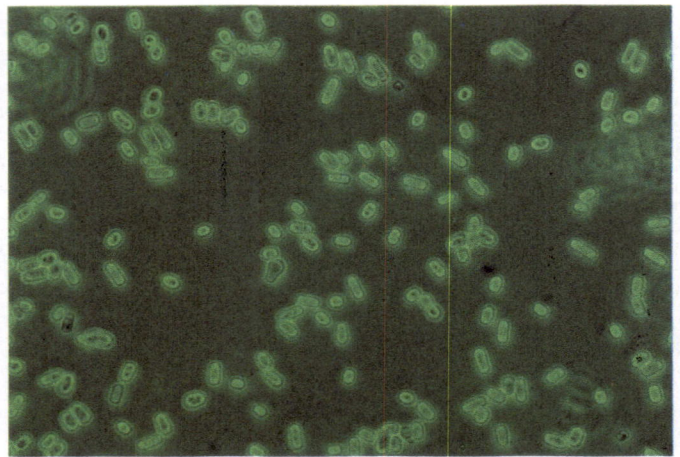

Fig. 81. *Geotrichum candidum.* Arthrospores in a wet preparation from Nervina agar (Grütz-III)

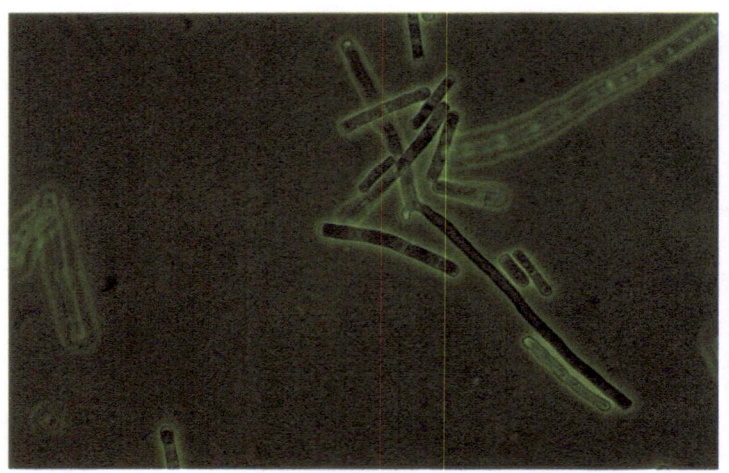

Fig. 82. *Geotrichum candidum.* Arthrospores and mycelia in a wet preparation from Nervina agar (Grütz-III)

116

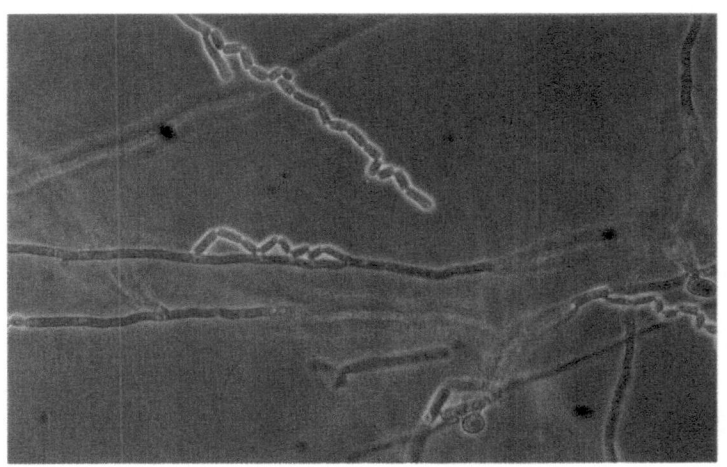

Fig. 83. *Geotrichum candidum* on rice agar (48 h). Mycelium and arthrospores

11.2 Fungal Cultures in Practice

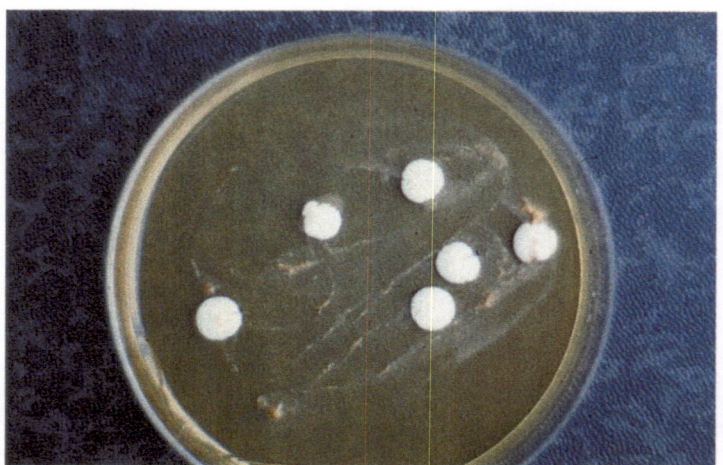

Fig. 84. Vaginal secretions on Nervina agar (Grütz-III). Isolated yeast colonies; asymptomatic colonization. *Candida* species, actual species not identified

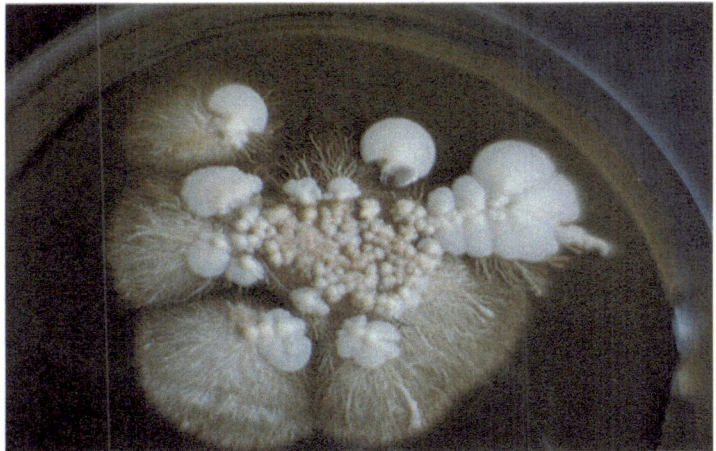

Fig. 85. Nervina agar (Grütz-III) with *Candida albicans,* cultured from vaginal secretions in a case of vaginal mycosis. After several days of growth, the vegetative mycelium of the yeast penetrates the agar. The surface of the colony remained smooth

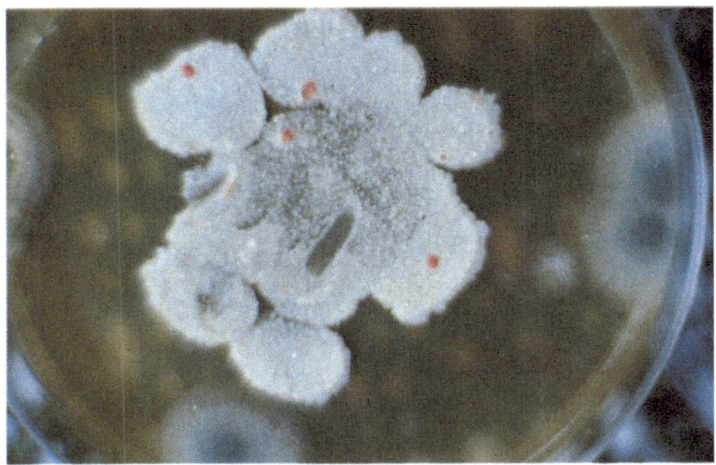

Fig. 86. Vaginal secretions on Nervina agar (Grütz-III) with yeast colonies. A mold at the periphery of the plate was an airborne contaminant. **White colonies;** species of *Candida,* probably *Candida albicans.* **Red colonies:** *Rhodotorula* species, probably *R. rubra*

119

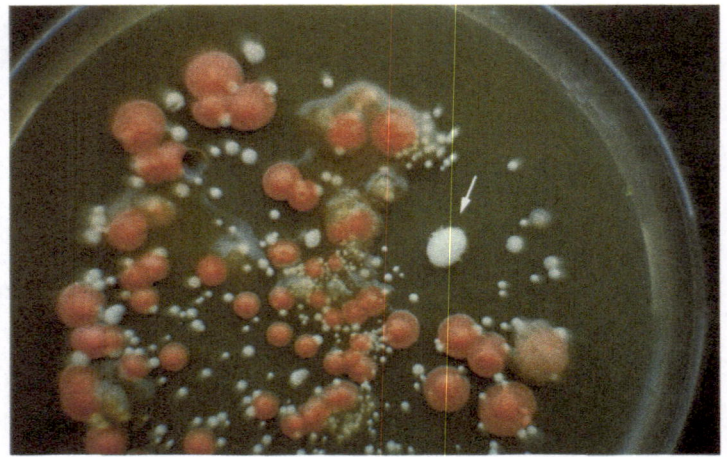

Fig. 87. Impression culture of erythematous apposed submammary skin regions (intertrigo) (Nervina agar Grütz-III). **Red:** *Rhodotorula rubra;* **yellow smears:** unidentified bacteria; **white:** small colonies: staphylococci, **white, large colony (arrow):** *Candida* sp

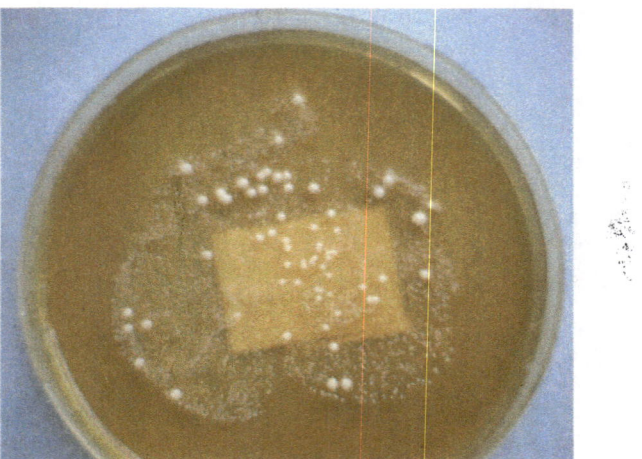

Fig. 88. Vaginal secretions on Nervina agar (Grütz-III). **Large colonies:** yeasts; **small colonies:** staphylococci

120

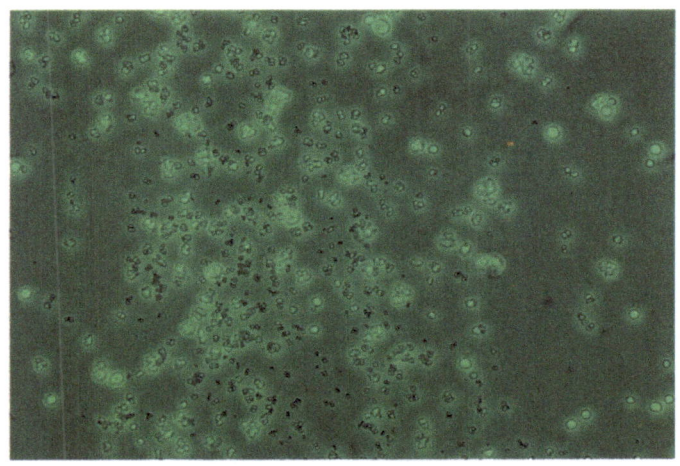

Fig. 89. Wet preparation from agar plate of Fig. 88. Budding cells and staphylococci, probably *Staphylococcus epidermidis*

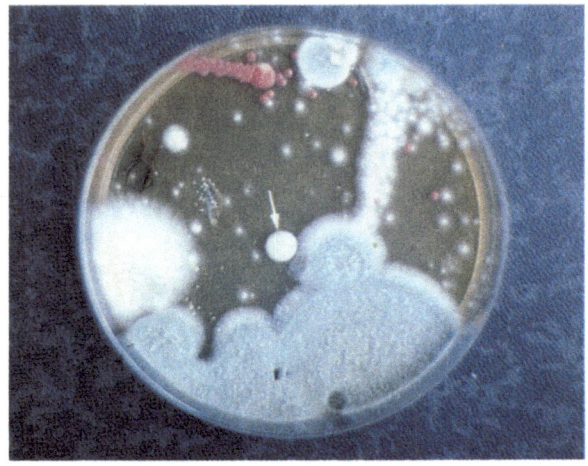

Fig. 90. Molds, *Rhodotorula rubra,* a *Candida* colony **(arrow)** and staphylococci growing on Nervina agar (Grütz-III)

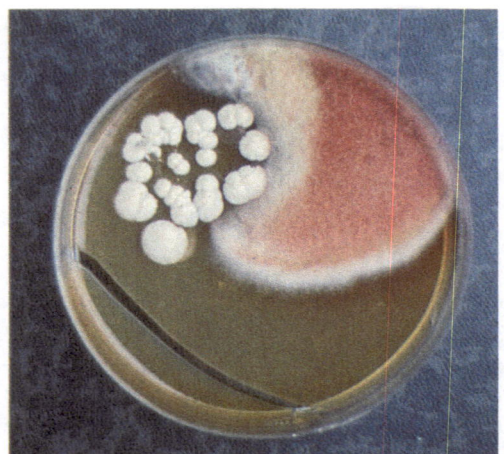

Fig. 91. Nervina agar (Grütz-III), fissured because of age and desiccation. Vaginal secretions. **White** colonies without aerial mycelium: yeasts, **white-and-red** with aerial mycelium: molds (airborne contaminants)

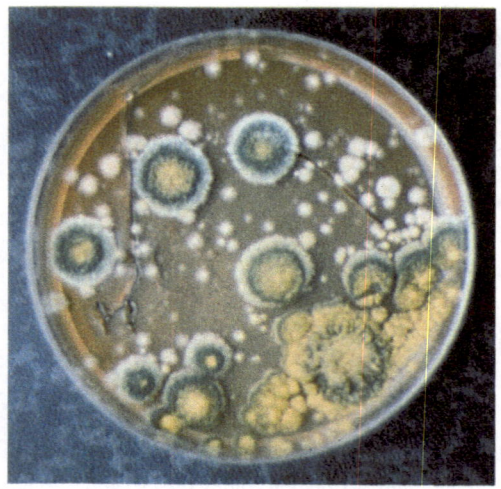

Fig. 92. Agar plate contaminated by molds

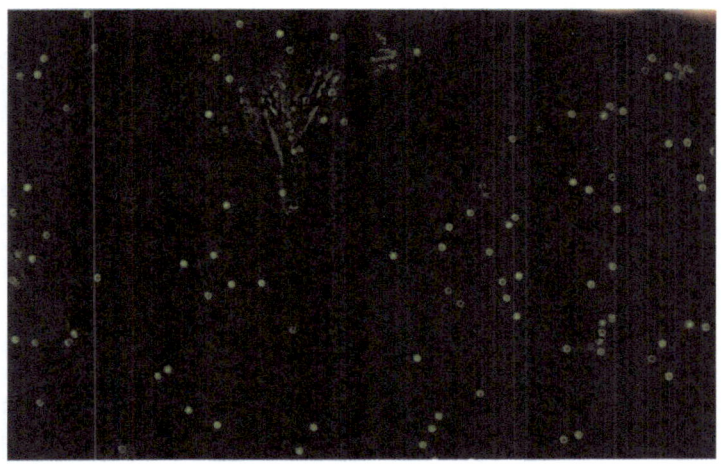

Fig. 93. Mold, *Penicillium* sp. Mycelium, conidiophore and conidia (spores)

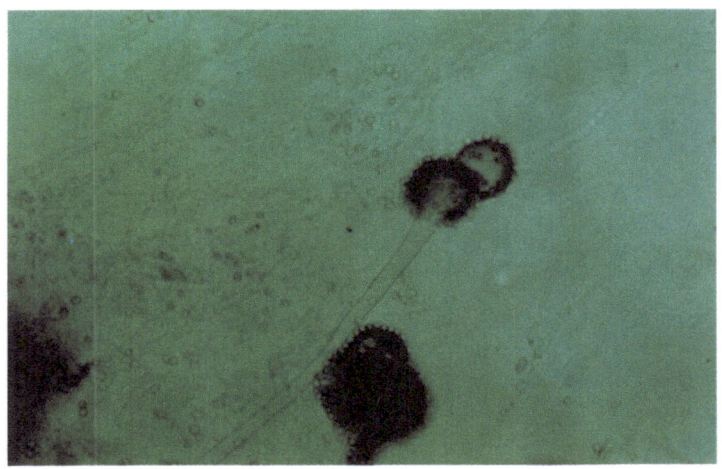

Fig. 94. Mold, *Aspergillus* sp. Mycelium, conidiophore with conidia (spores)

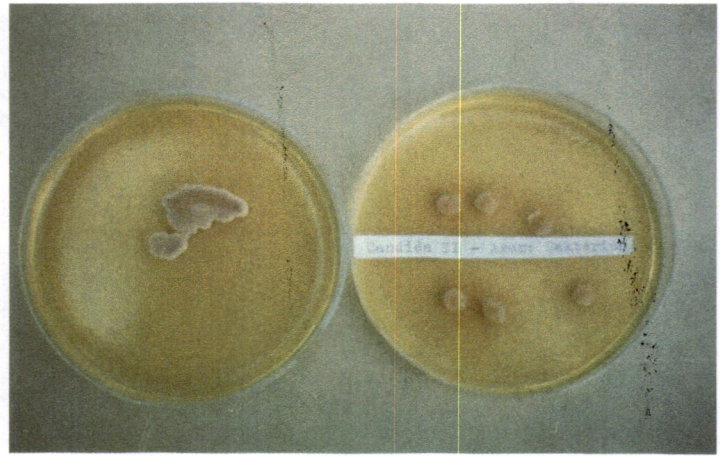

Fig. 95. Candida-II agar. **Left:** *Candida albicans,* **right:** bacteria. Both isolates from vaginal secretions. Bacteria rarely grow on this agar

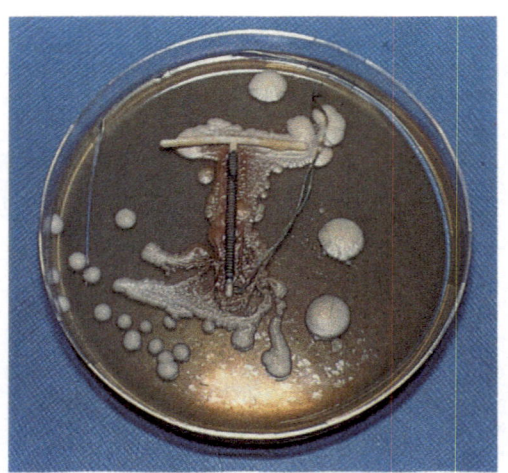

Fig. 96. The demonstration of yeasts on the T portion of an IUD does not necessarily mean that yeasts are adhering intrauterine surface. On being drawn out, the entire device is contaminated by the yeasts colonizing the external os

11.3 Suitability Testing of Nickerson's Agar

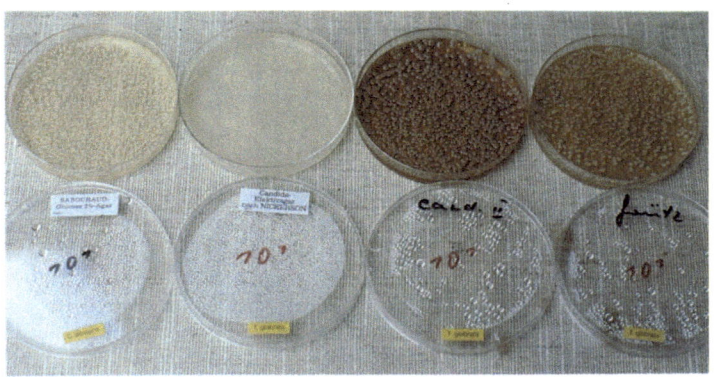

Fig. 97. *Candida albicans* on Sabouraud's 2% dextrose agar **(left)** and *Candida glabrata* on Nickerson's agar, Candida-II agar and Nervina agar (Grütz III), 10^1 cells/ml in saline, 0.4 ml per plate. Growth on all media except Nickerson's agar

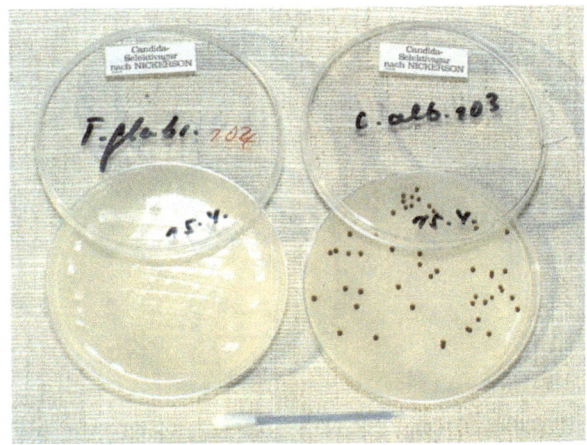

Fig. 98. Material from a suspension of yeast cells in saline was streaked on Nickerson's agar with a swab of cotton wool. **Left:** 10^4 cells/ml were not sufficient to obtain a positive result with *Candida glabrata*. **Right:** colonies of *Candida albicans* grew from a suspension of only 10^3 cells/ml

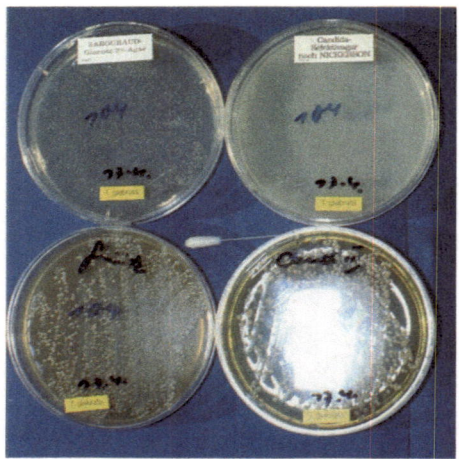

Fig. 99. *Candida glabrata*, 10^4 cells/ml in saline, applied with a cotton wool swab to Sabouraud's 2% glucose agar, Nickerson's agar, Nervina agar-Grütz III and Candida-II agar. No growth on Nickerson's agar

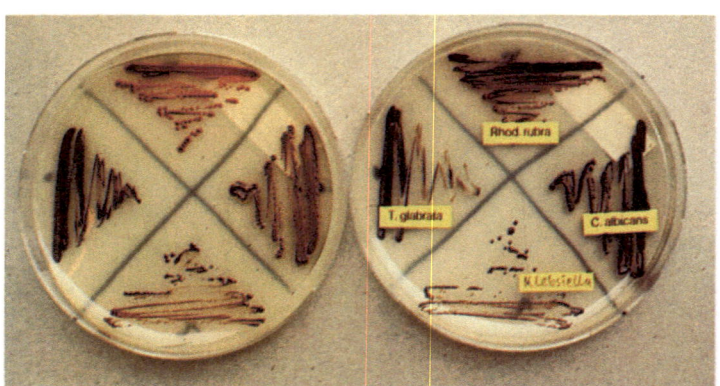

Fig. 100. Examples of Nickerson's agar by the same manufacturer but different batches; identical inoculations. **Right:** *Rhodotorula rubra* was not identified because it lacked the red color; brown colonies were also formed by bacteria (in this case *Klebsiella*; also *E.coli*, staphylococci etc.); *Candida glabrata*, with a low cell count produced poor growth (towards the centre of the loop mark). Odor atypical even of *Candida* spp

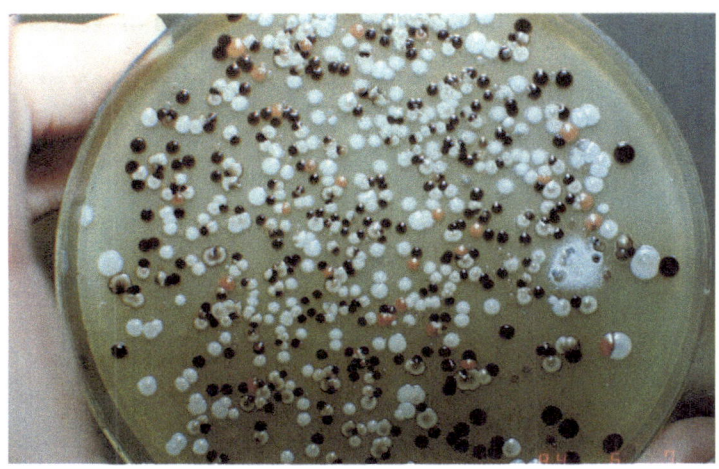

Fig. 101. Experimentally contamined urine sample on Nickerson's agar. *Rhodotorula rubra* **(red),** *Candida* species **(white),** bacteria **(brown),** molds **(greenish)**

11.4 Some Methods for the Differentiation of Yeasts

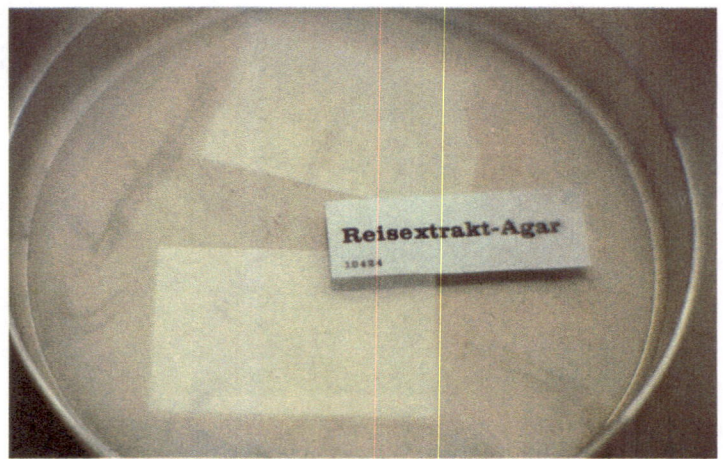

Fig. 102. Rice extract agar. Plate inoculated with a yeast. Cover slip in place, room temperature

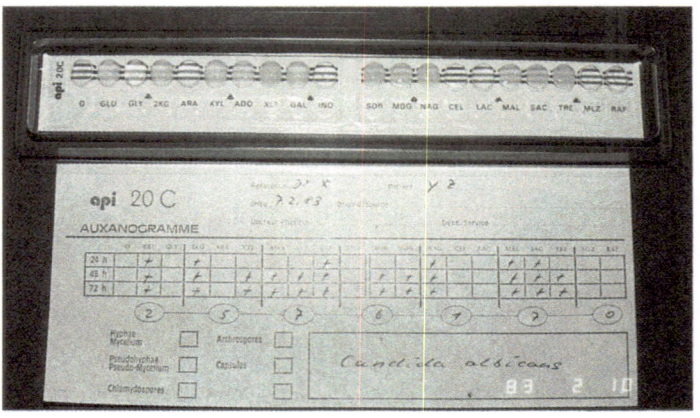

Fig. 103. Yeasts can usually be reliably identified by a combination of morphological and biochemical characteristics. Above: *Candida albicans*, identification by means of the API 20 C Auxanogramme System (API System S.A., La Balme Les Grottes, F-38390 Montalien Vercien, France)

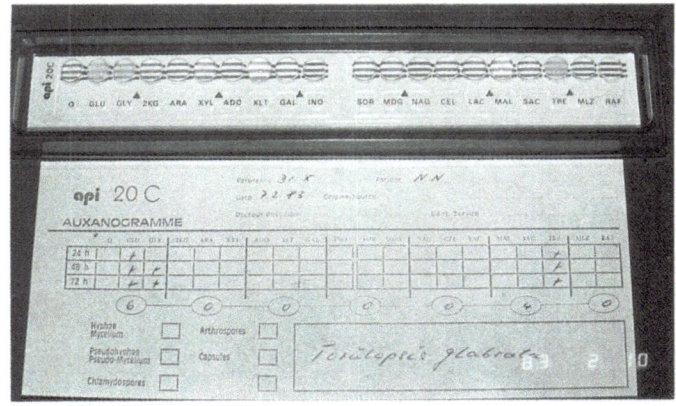

Fig. 104. Identification of *Candida glabrata* with the Api 20 C Auxano-gramme System

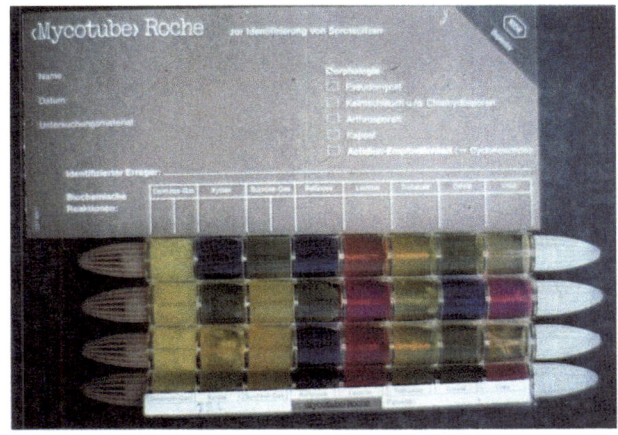

Fig. 105. Identification of *Candida* spp. with the aid of the Mycotube Roche system (Hoffmann-La Roche)

11.5 Wet Preparations from Vaginal Secretions

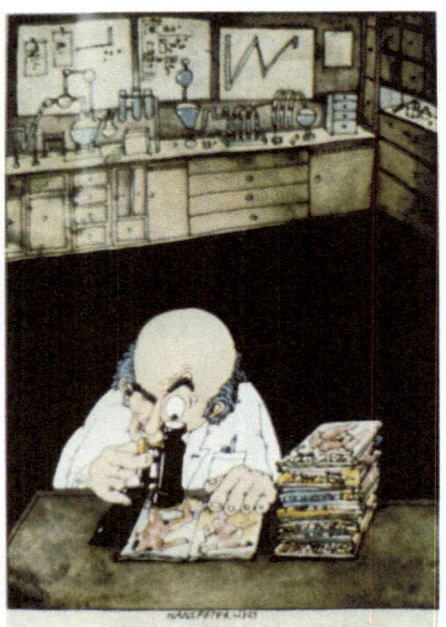

Fig. 106. A wet preparation (from Penthouse)

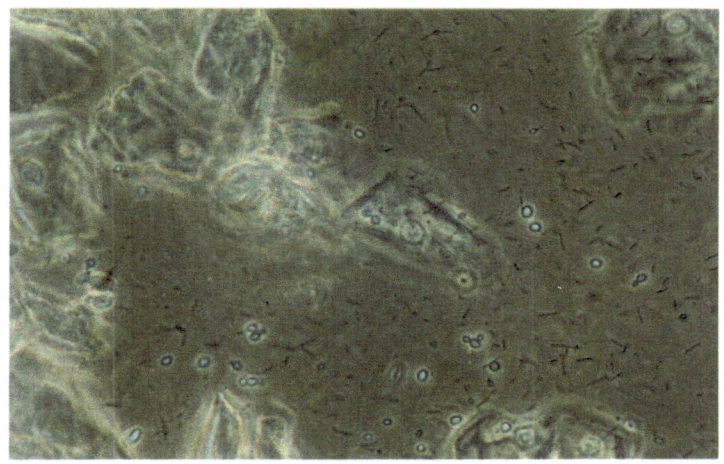

Fig. 107. Wet preparation from vaginal secretions. Döderlein flora and (exceptional numbers of) budding cells, probably *Candida (Torulopsis) glabrata*. No signs of infection

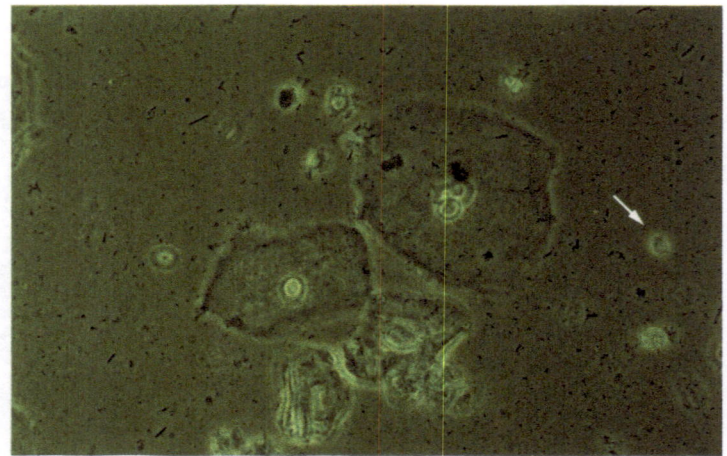

Fig. 108. Wet preparation from vaginal secretions in bacterial vaginosis; the single budding cell **(arrow)** is easy to miss. No clinical signs of candidosis

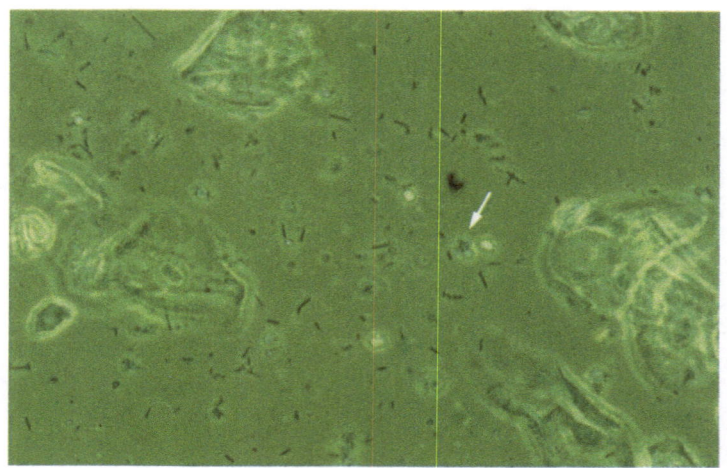

Fig. 109. Wet preparation from vaginal secretions in a case of vaginal candidosis. Lactobacilli, two yeast cells one over the other, one of them budding **(arrow)**

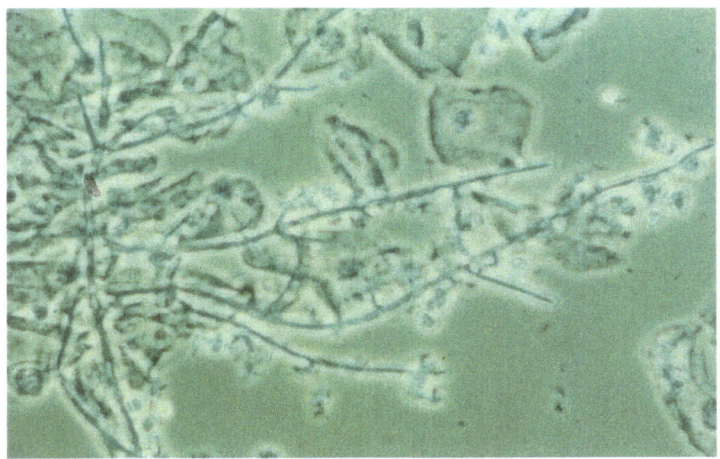

Fig. 110. Copious pseucomycelium in a wet preparation of vaginal secretions in vaginal candidosis in pregnancy

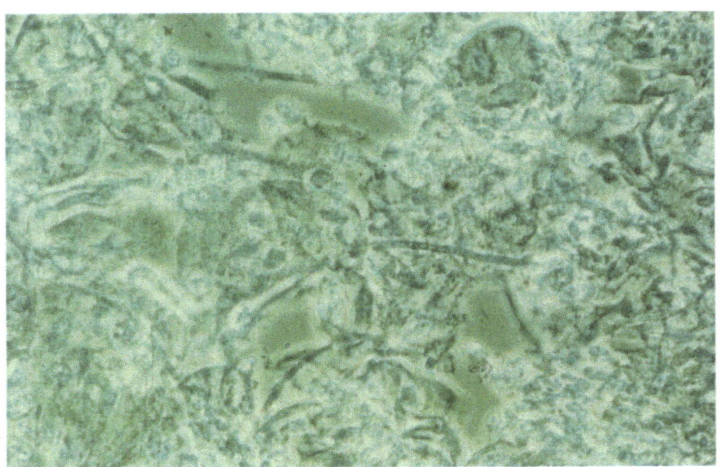

Fig. 111. Wet preparation from vaginal secretions in vaginal candidosis. The pseudohyphae may be missed in the (too) dense conglomeration of cells. KOH may be useful in such cases

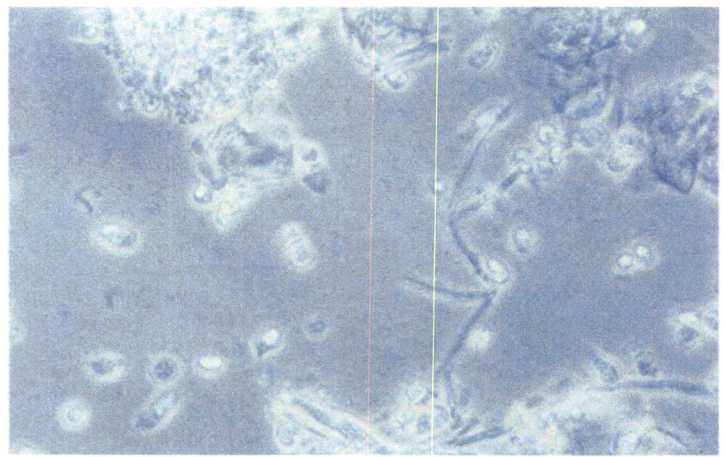

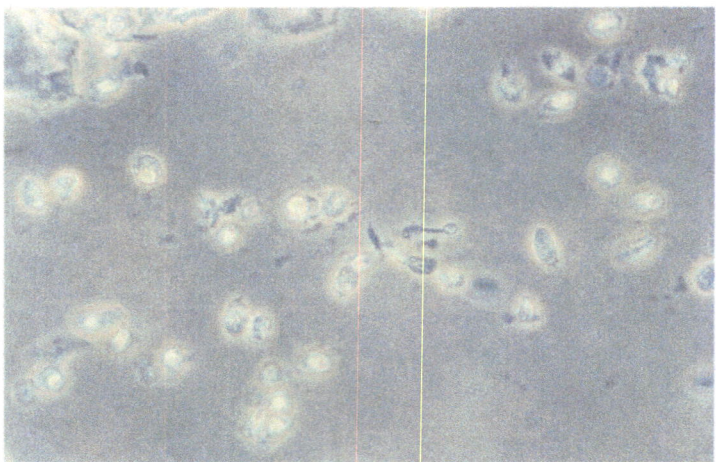

Fig. 112, 113. Wet preparation from vaginal secretions in acute vaginal candidosis caused by *Candida albicans*. **Fig. 112.** Pseudohyphae and many leukocytes, few bacteria. **Fig. 113.** Budding cell and small pseudomycelium. Underneath, a leukocyte with a partially intercellular portion of pseudomycelium

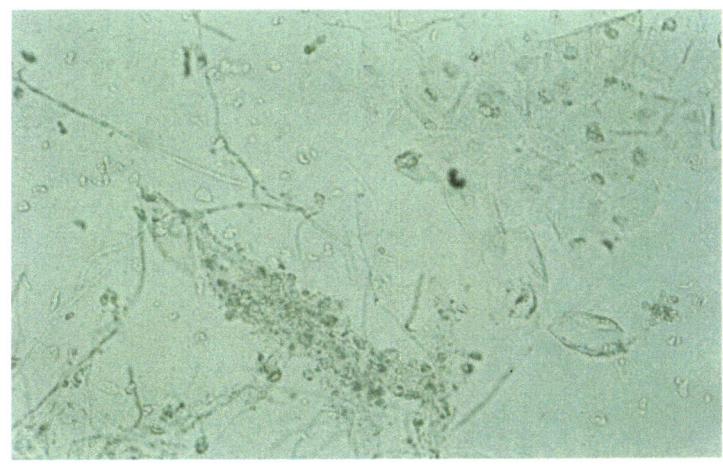

Fig. 114. Wet preparation from vaginal secretions in vaginal candidosis. Branched pseudomycelium. Bright-ground microscopy is less three-dimensional than phase-contrast microscopy

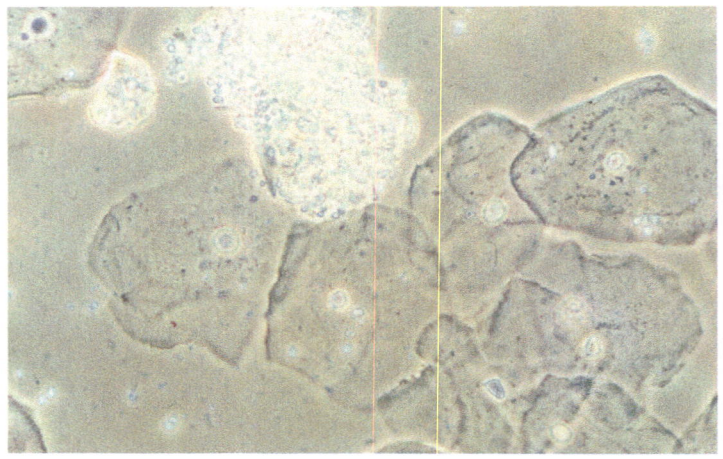

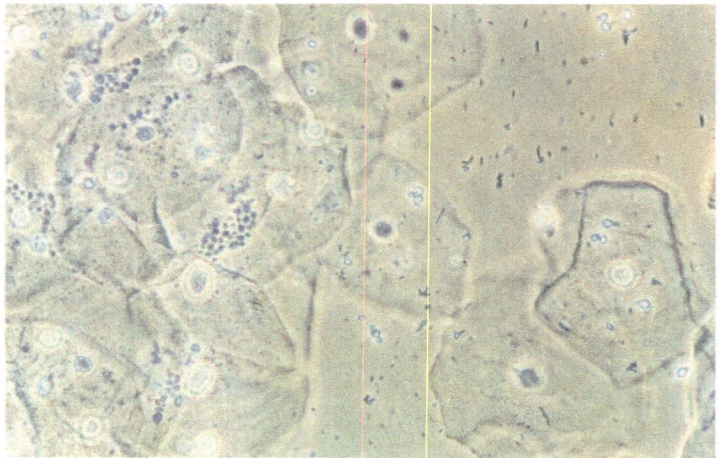

Fig. 115, 116. Wet preparation from vaginal secretions in a case of vaginal complaints, caused by *Candida glabrata,* that had been recurring for years. **Fig. 115.** Conglomerate of budding cells. **Fig. 116.** Apparently budding cells of dark appearance adhering to vaginal epithelial cells, light budding cells free in the secretions

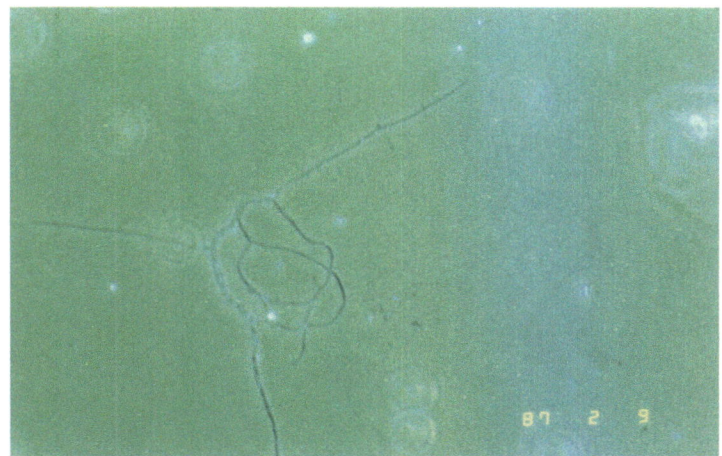

Fig. 117. Hyphae of molds in a wet preparation of a vaginal secretions. However, the fungi emanated from a saline solution that had not been renewed for weeks!

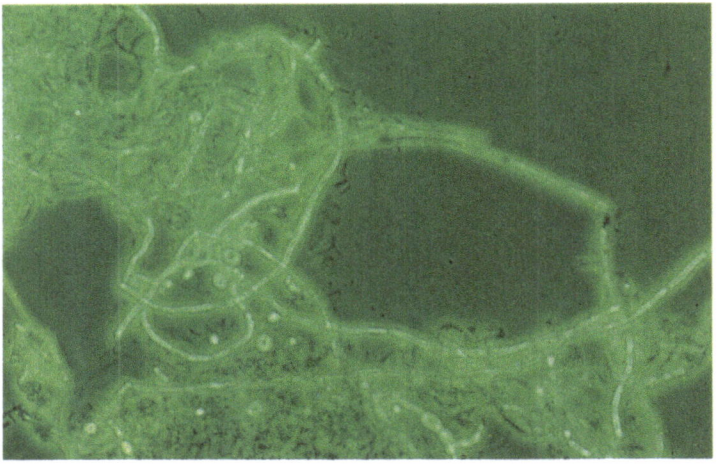

Fig. 118. Cotton wool fibres – not hyphae!

11.6 Cytology and Histology

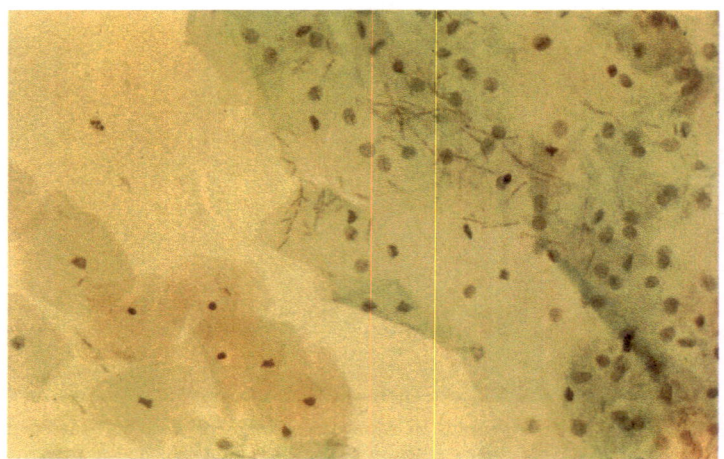

Fig. 119. Papanicolaou's cytological smear test, showing pseudohyphae

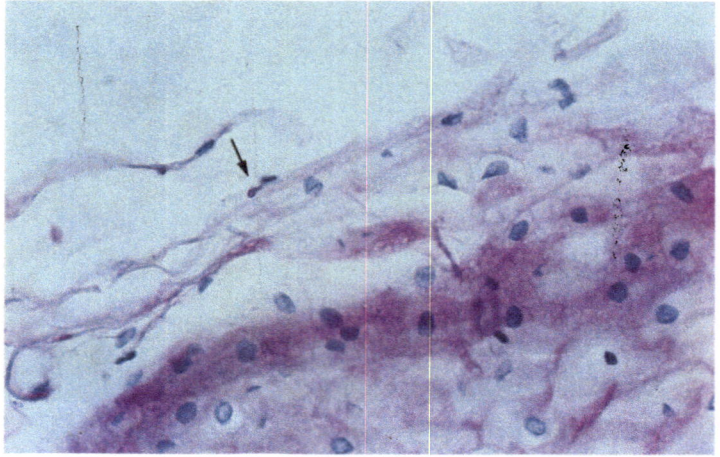

Fig. 120. Histological section of the vaginal wall in vaginal mycosis, culture yielded *Candida albicans*. Only one blastospore discernible **(arrow)**, (H and E stain, × 400)

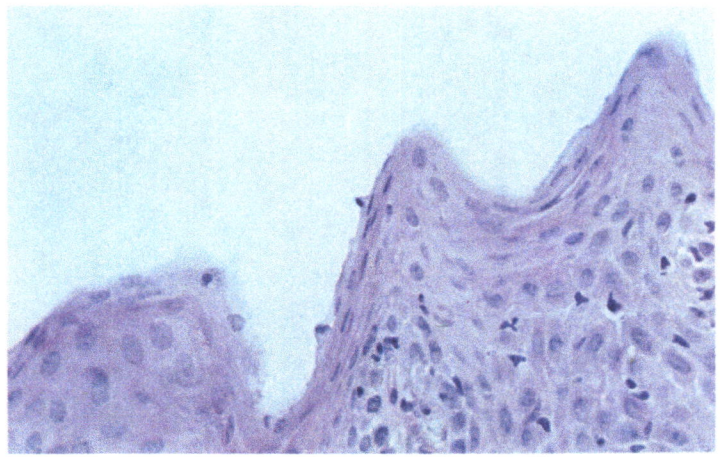

Fig. 121. Histological section of the vaginal wall in a case of very severe vulvovaginal mycosis, culture: *Candida albicans*. The plate shows no yeasts (H and E stain, × 400)

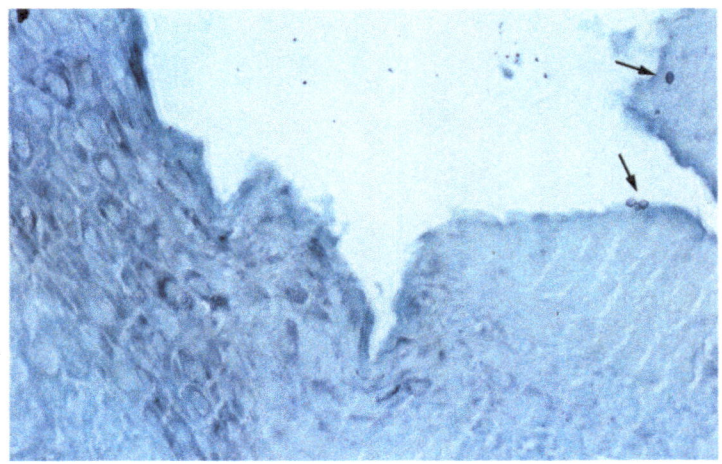

Fig. 122. Histological section of the vaginal wall in recurrent mycosis causing mild symptoms. Culture: *Candida glabrata*. No signs of inflammation, isolated budding cells **(arrows)** (Grocott's stain, × 400)

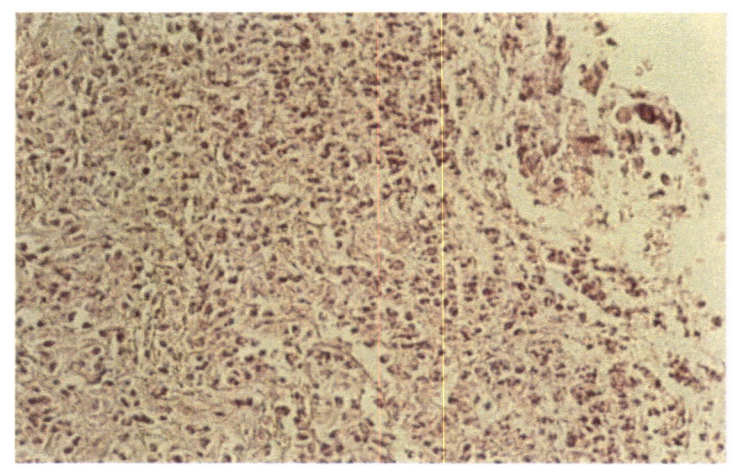

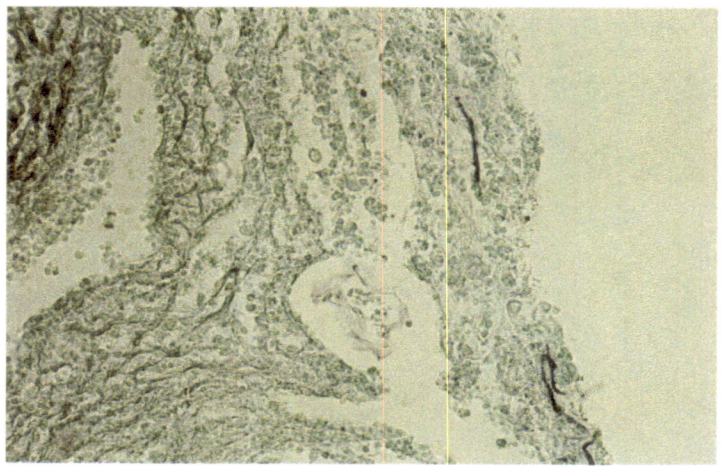

Fig. 123, 124*

* The preparations are from a study carried out jointly with Dr. M. Günther, Institut für Pathologie der Stadt Wuppertal (Director: Prof. Dr. med. G. E. Schubert).

11.7 Clinical Pictures

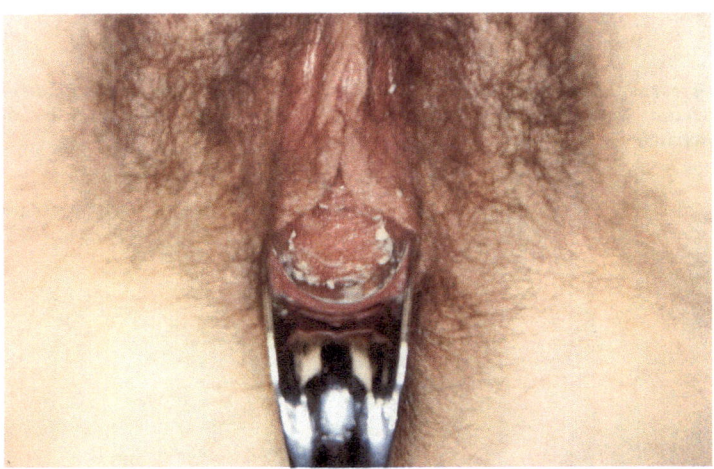

Fig. 125. Typical appearance of an acute vaginal candidosis (culture: *Candida albicans*) in the 14th week of pregnancy

◄──

Fig. 123, 124 . Histological section of the lower urethra in a woman (died aged 79) with diabetes mellitus, kidney failure, myocardial infarction and urogenital candidosis (culture: *Candida albicans*). **Fig. 123.** H and E stain. No fungal elements discernible in this case of severe hemorrhagic urethritis. **Fig. 124.** Grocott's stain. Visualization of pseudohyphae indicating mycosis

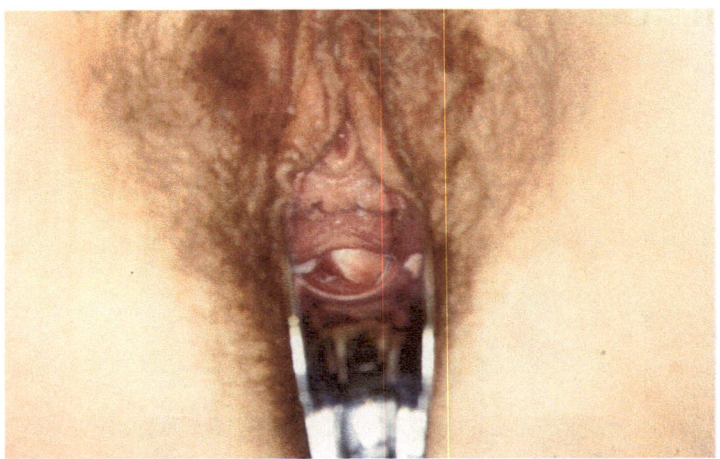

Fig. 126. Occasional mild burning for the last 4 years; culture: *Candida glabrata*. Typically: slight reddening, usually scanty, grey non-offensive discharge

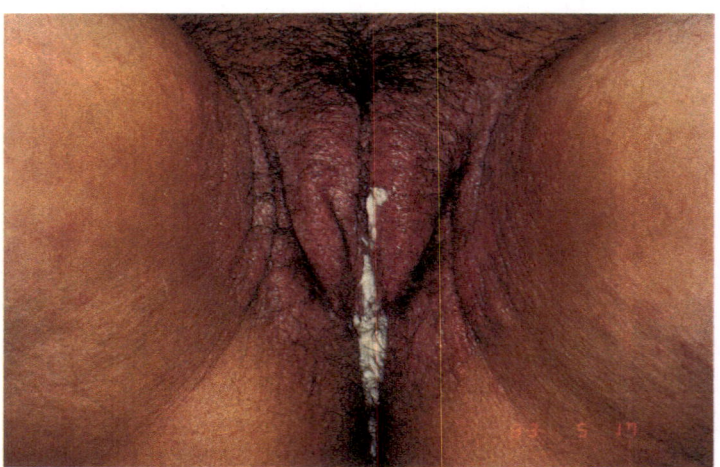

Fig. 127. Severe vulvovaginitis "suffered" for a period of several weeks. Pathogen: *Candida albicans*. Third trimester of pregnancy. Partly vesicular, partly follicular cutaneous candidosis of the vulva and thighs

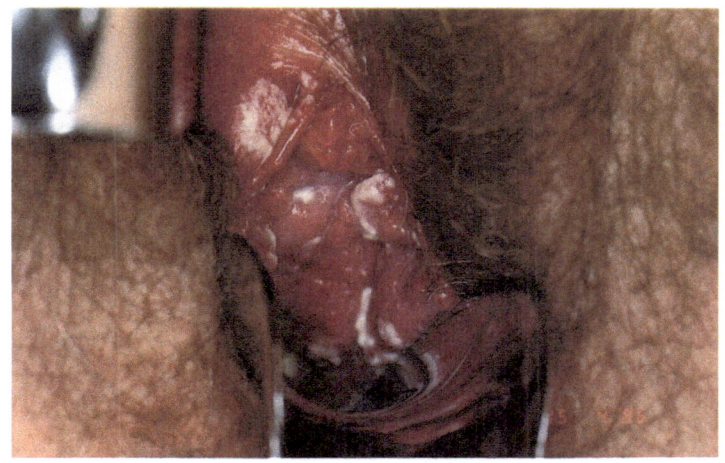

Fig. 128. Vulvovaginal mycosis *(Candida albicans)* with fungal plaques that could not be wiped off

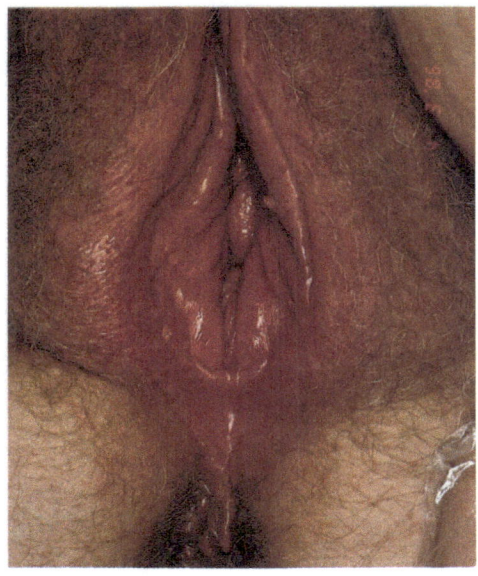

Fig. 129. Vulvovaginal mycosis *(Candida albicans)* with epithelial lesions in the region of the posterior commissure

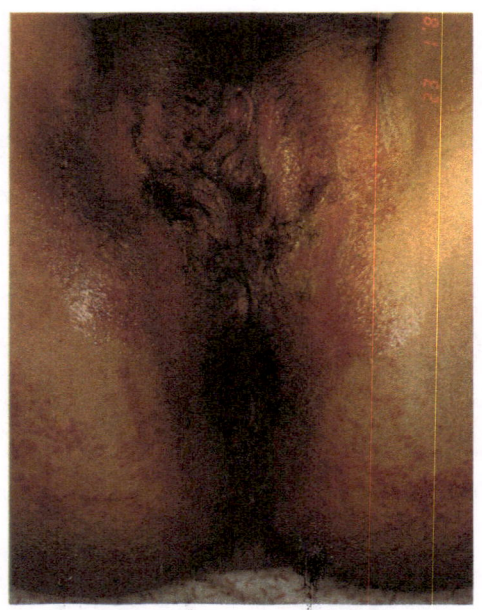

Fig. 130–133. Young woman with severe vulvocandidosis *(Candida albicans)*. Partly vesicular, partly eczematous form; erosions.

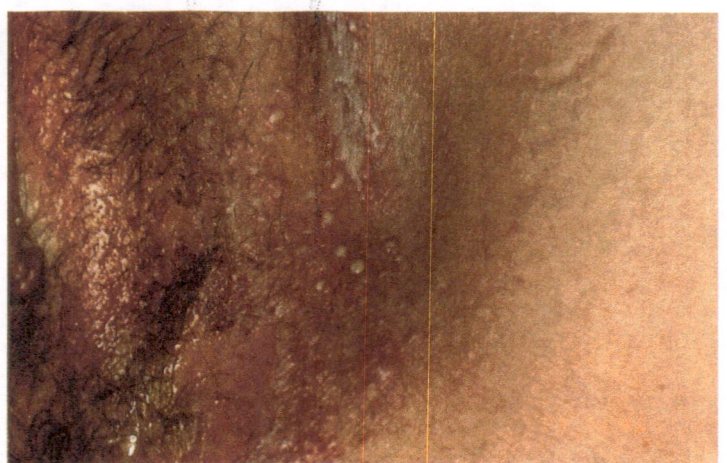

Fig. 131

144

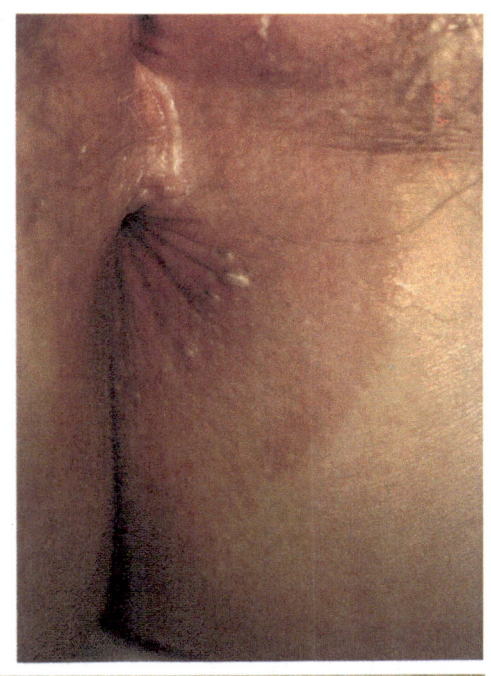

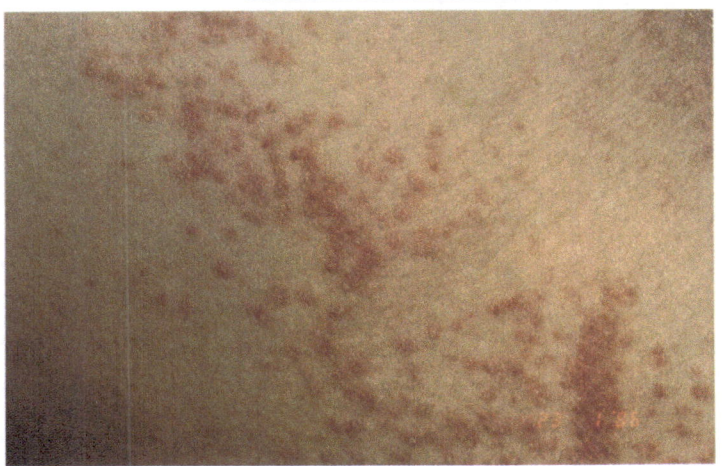

Fig. 132, 133

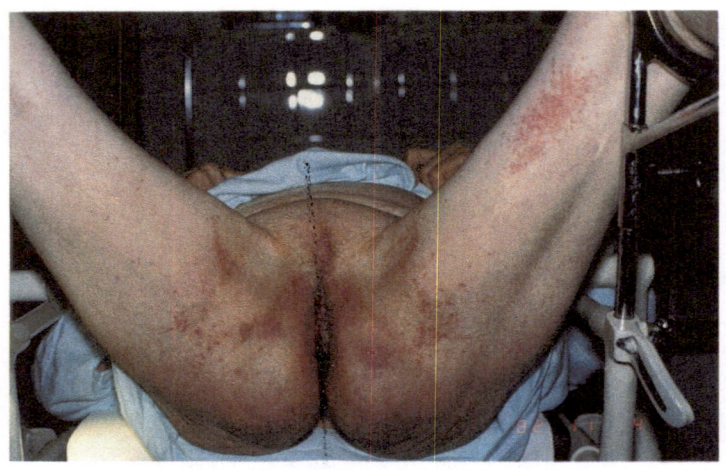

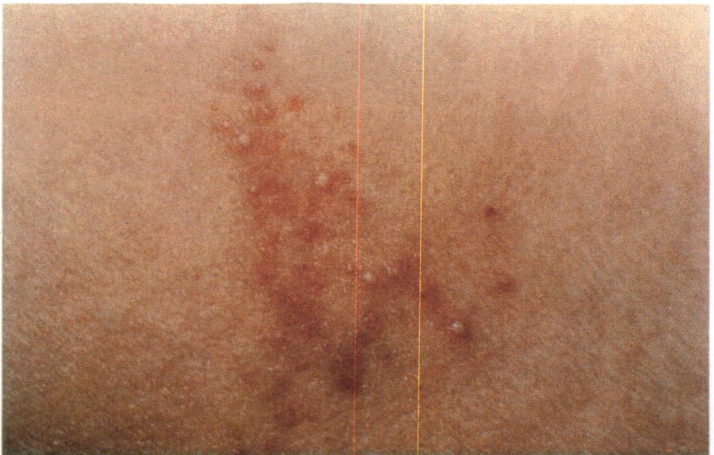

Fig. 134, 135. 81-year old patient, condition after "minor" vulvectomy approx. 10 days previously, perioperative prophylactic antibiotic treatment given. Vesicular form of candidosis on the thighs emanating from a vaginal yeast colonization (*Candida albicans* cultured from the vagina and from vesicles)

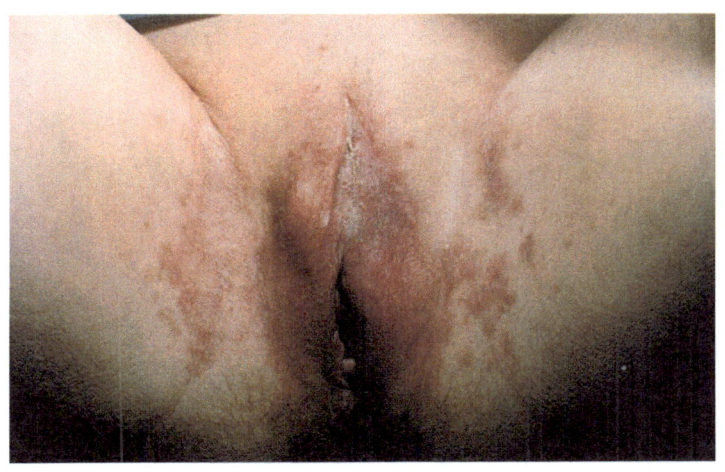

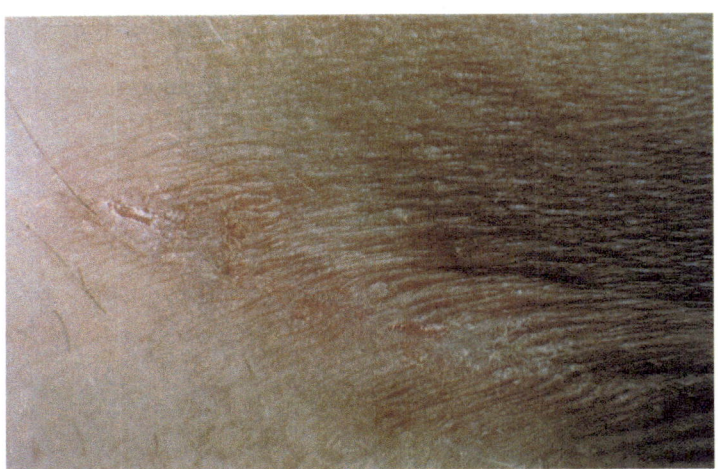

Fig. 136, 137. Patient, 45 years, condition after partial vulvectomy for amelanotic melanoma. Eczematous form of vulvocandidosis

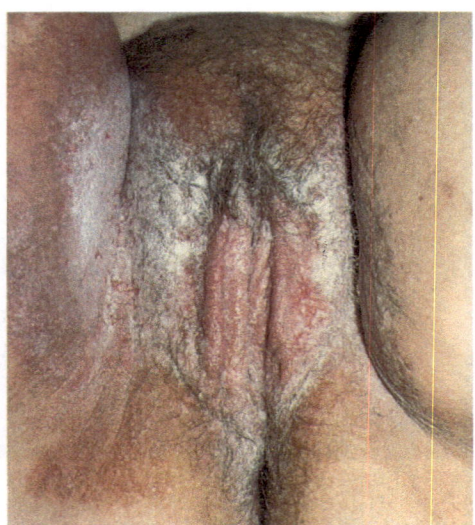

Fig. 138. Severely obese patient, 50 years, burning of the vulva for the last 4 weeks, had treated herself with "Penatencreme" (skin cream). Culture: *Candida albicans*

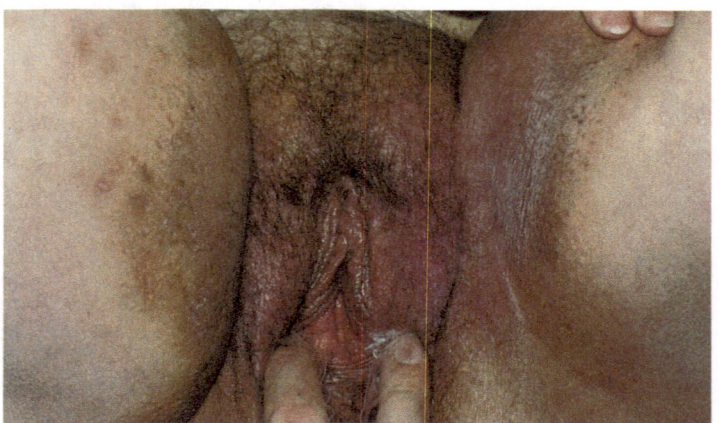

Fig. 139. After two weeks of topical treatment with cream (and vaginal tablets), marked improvement in the candidosis but incomplete subsidence of the symptoms despite a negative fungal culture. Obvious reddening of the vulva and groins and small fissures. Intolerance of an intimate hygiene lotion. It is likely that the candidal invasion was secondary to the skin irritation

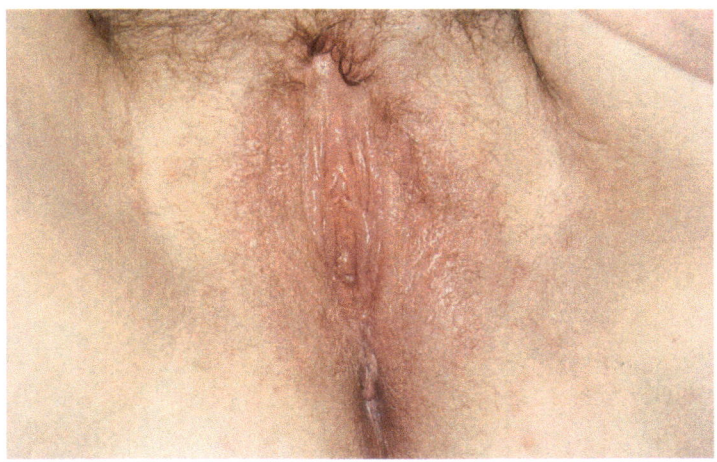

Fig. 140. 20-year old, 4 weeks post partum, erosive vulvitis causing distressing burning. Culture of *Candida glabrata* despite two weeks of antifungal treatment but no mycosis. Microbial eczema. Symptoms and signs subsided in response to an antibiotic-corticosteroid ointment

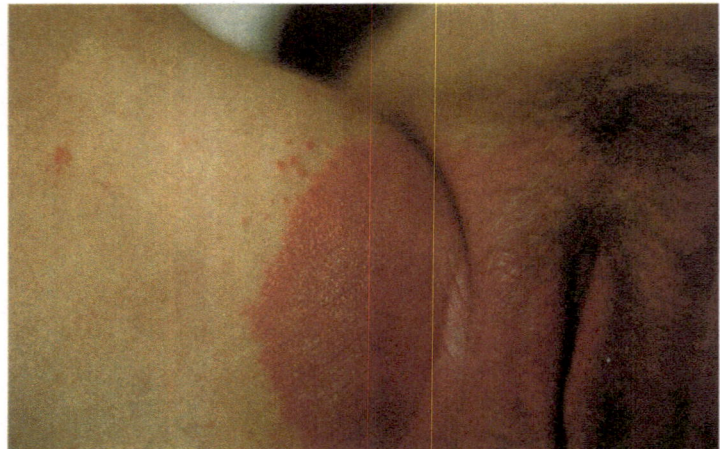

Fig. 141. Neurodermatitis circumscripta of the vulva in a 74-year old patient currently undergoing radiotherapy for cervical carcinoma. The culturally demonstrated yeasts *(Candida glabrata)* in the vagina have no relevance to the clinical picture. The diagnosis was made only when the yeast had been eliminated with antifungal agents without any change in the signs or symptoms

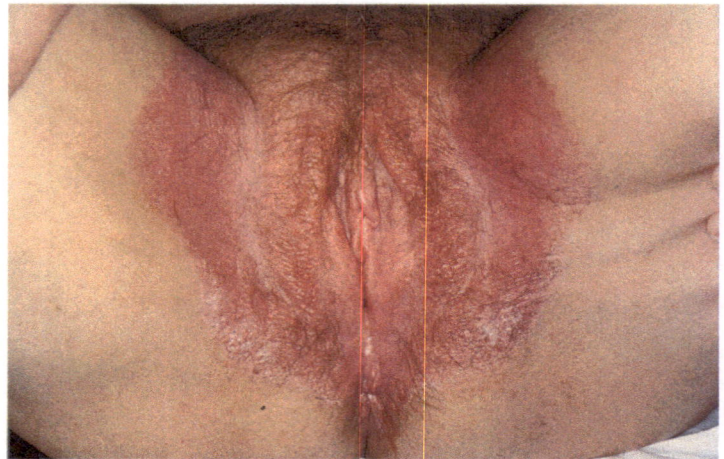

Fig. 142. The same patient approx. 1 year later. She had seen no physician in the interval. The fungal culture was now negative

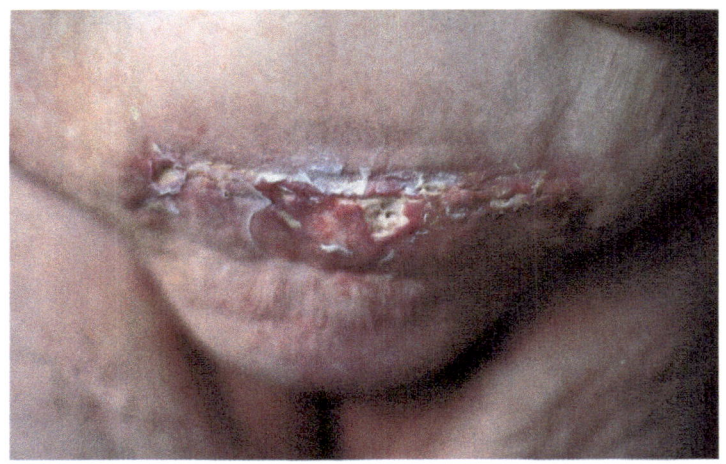

Fig. 143. Laparotomy wound in incurable ovarian carcinoma. Superinfection of the wound with *Candida albicans*

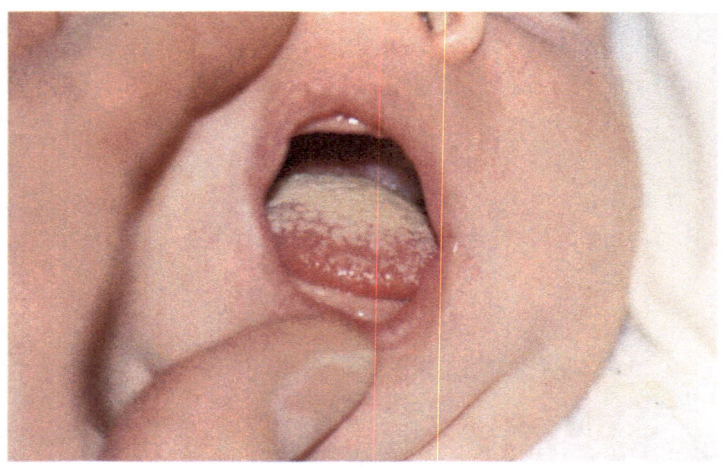

Fig. 144. Oral "thrush" in a 4 week old infant (culture: *Candida albicans*)

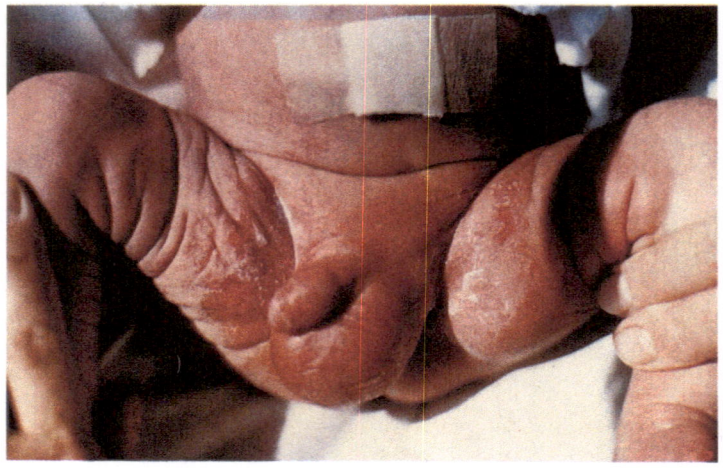

Fig. 145. Mycosis caused by *Candida albicans* in an infant aged a few days ("diaper" or "napkin-area dermatitis")

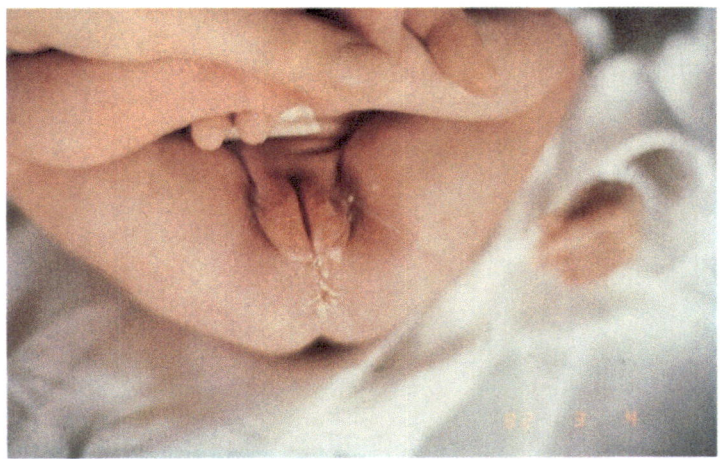

Fig. 146. Early stage of candidosis in an infant aged a few days (the vulva is reddened and sore)

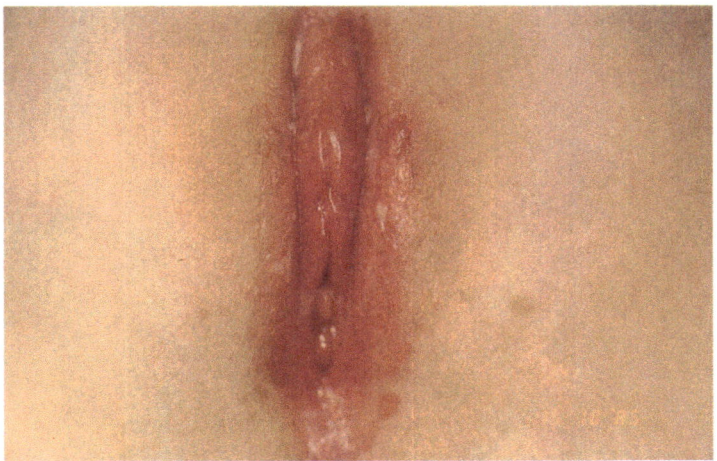

Fig. 147. 7 year old child treated by the pediatrician with oral trimethoprim + sulfamethoxazole for redness and burning of the vulva. Culture: *Candida albicans*. The candidosis cleared up in this otherwise healthy child in response to a single dose of clotrimazole 10% vaginal cream and a 6-day treatment of the vulva with clotrimazole 1% cream

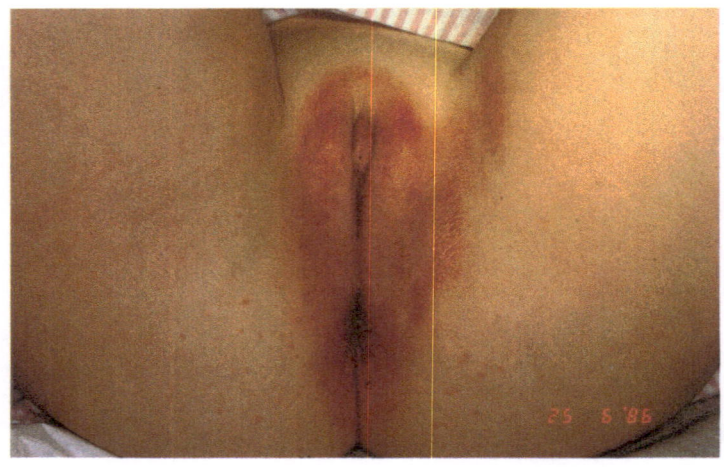

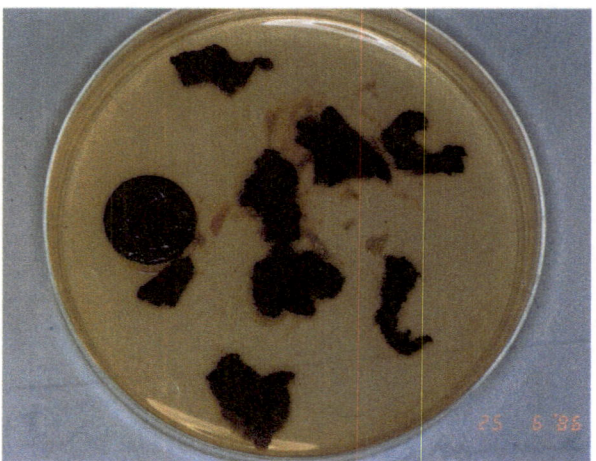

Fig. 148, 149. 4-year old girl; increasingly severe vulvitis for 7 weeks. This began with a discharge which became watery and foul. Pediatric treatment with nonspecific baths for suspected bacterial or fungal vulvitis. The **diagnosis** was made after vaginoscopy: intravaginal foreign bodies (a Pfennig coin and pieces of foam stuffing from a teddy bear) with vulvovaginitis. Fungal culture negative

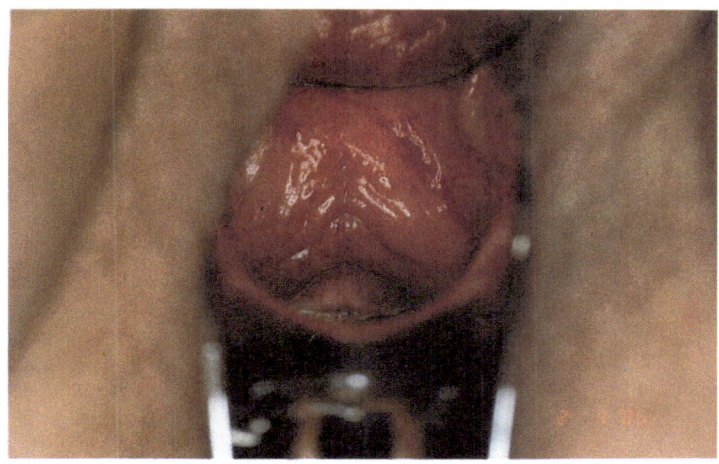

Fig. 150. The patient, aged 55 years, presented herself for a routine smear test without complaining of symptoms. Sparse yellowish-green discharge. Patchy red lesions of the vagina, petechiae on contact of the speculum. Wet preparation: leukocytes, coccoid bacteria, fungal culture as well as enzymatic immunoassays for chlamydia and gonococci negative. **Diagnosis:** bacterial colpitis – by contrast with bacterial vaginosis and vaginal mycosis this is a rare condition, possibly combined with hormone deficiency

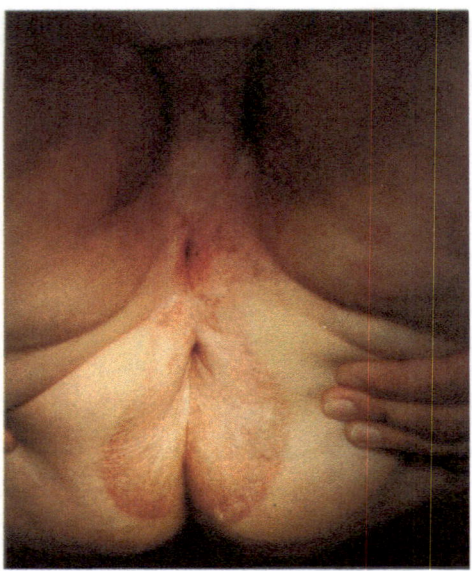

Fig. 151. 75-year old patient, condition after vulvectomy several years ago. Pruritus in the vulvar region for some time, non-itching perianal lesion with raised margins. **Diagnosis:** lichen sclerosus of the vulva, perianal psoriasis (only one visible lesion at the present time)

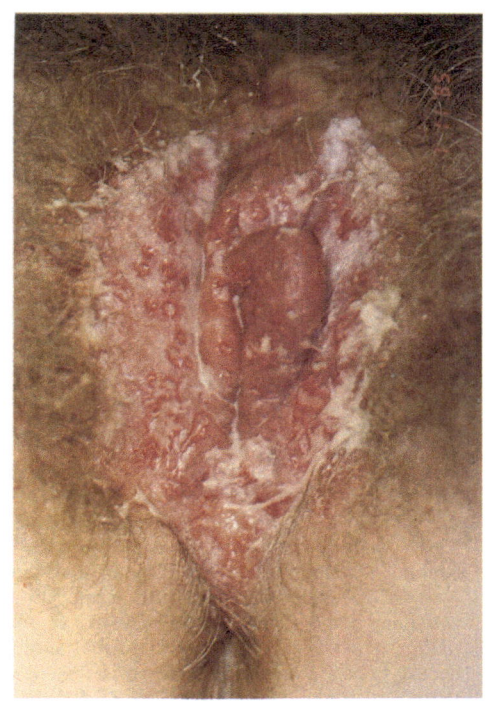

Fig. 152. 18-year old patient, severe pain in the vulva for 3 days, swelling of the lymph nodes in both groins and initial pyrexia: typical picture of a primary herpes infection. Because of an initially positive fungal culture, the patient was admitted for "refractory vaginal mycosis"

157

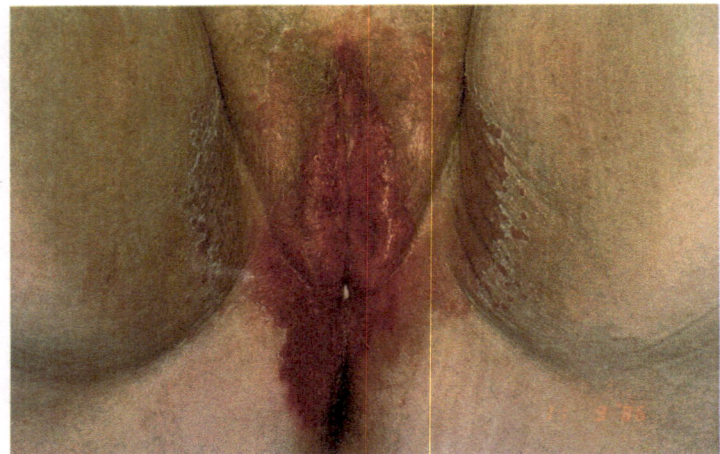

Fig. 153. 54-year old patient*, operation in 1979 for carcinoma of the corpus uteri, 1980: extirpation of a vaginal recurrence, 1981 radiotherapy for a further vaginal recurrence, from 1982 onwards itching and burning of the vagina; since then, according to the patient, she had been treated by a gynecologist and a dermatologist with about 30 different ointments. From approximately the spring of 1986 onwards, very severe discomfort during urination, when sitting etc. Topical corticosteroids, hormones and antifungal agents provided no relief. **Diagnosis:** extensive carcinoma *in situ* of the vulva and vagina (formerly called Paget's disease), extensive vulvovaginal candidosis (culture: *Candida albicans*)

---

* I take this opportunity of thanking Professor Dr. med. E. Haneke, Director of the Hautklinik der Ferdinand-Sauerbruch-Kliniken Wuppertal-Elberfeld, for the referral of this patient.

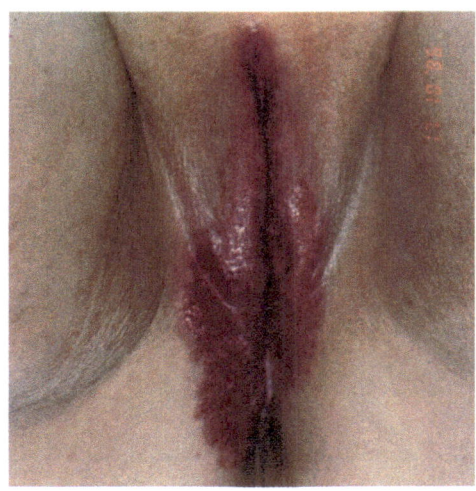

Fig. 154. The same patient (Fig. 153) after consistent topical and (because of pain on application of the cream) oral treatment of the candidosis. There remained the sharply marginated carcinoma *in situ* which was later extirpated by vulvectomy

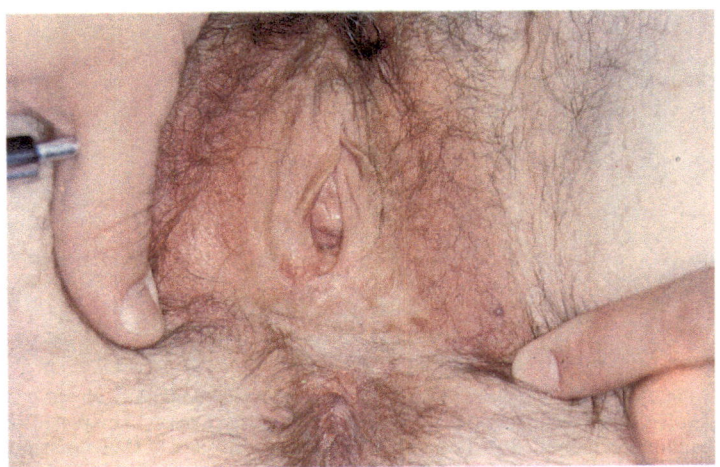

Fig. 155. Repeated treatment for "recurrent fungal infections" and pruritus of the vulva. **Diagnosis:** carcinoma in *situ* of the vulva (Bowen's disease)

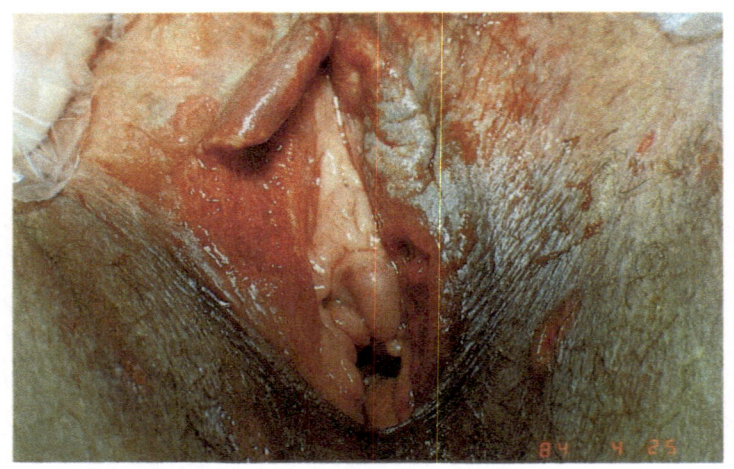

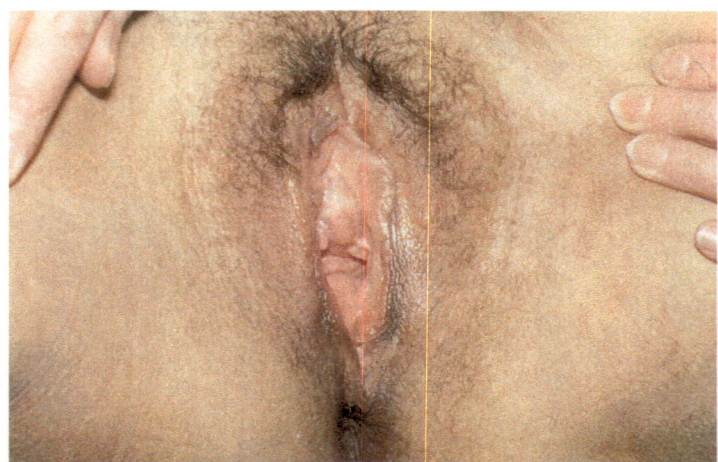

Fig. 156, 157. Patient, 30 years old, acute onset of painful ulcers of the vulva. A gynecologist in practice also demonstrated yeasts. The patient was ultimately admitted to hospital for "refractory mycosis". **Diagnosis:** probably Behçet's syndrome but possibly ulcus vulvae acutum (Lipschütz's ulcer) after herpes genitalis, chancroid and syphilis were ruled out. The condition cleared up spontaneously after 5 weeks, leaving labial defects **(Fig. 157)**

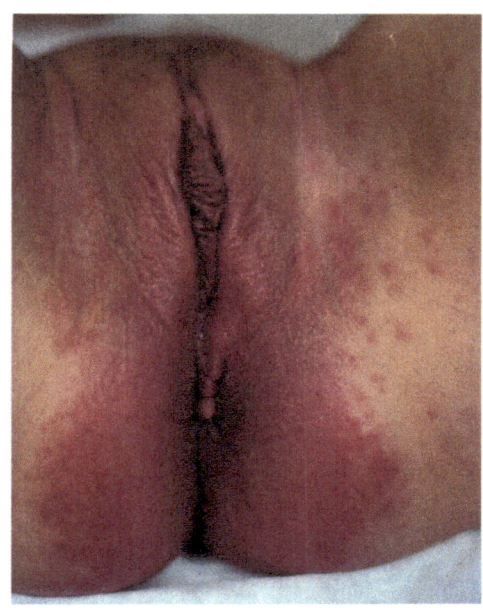

Fig. 158. 26-year old patient allergic to local anesthetics contained in an ointment for the relief of hemorrhoids which she had used without the knowledge of her physician while being treated for infections with trichomonads and yeasts. A deterioration in the area locally prompted thoughts of "resistance to treatment" or "allergy to clotrimazole"

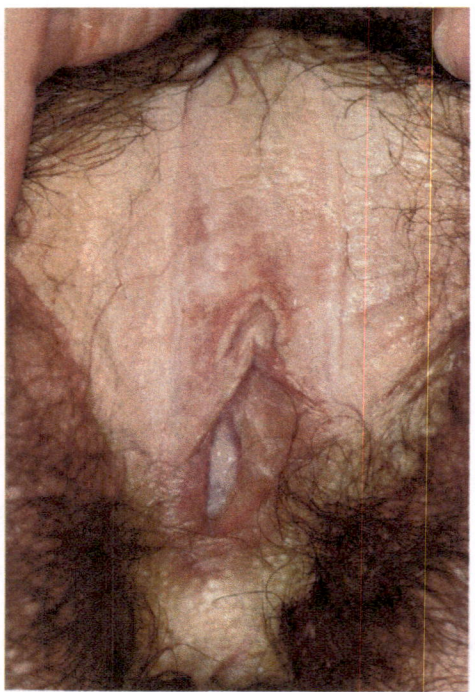

Fig. 159. 15-year old with anorexia nervosa and secondary amenorrhea. Pruritus of the vulva for some time to which she admitted only in answer to a direct question. ("well yes, I've always got fungi there and once I was given an ointment but it didn't do any good"). **Diagnosis:** lichen sclerosus

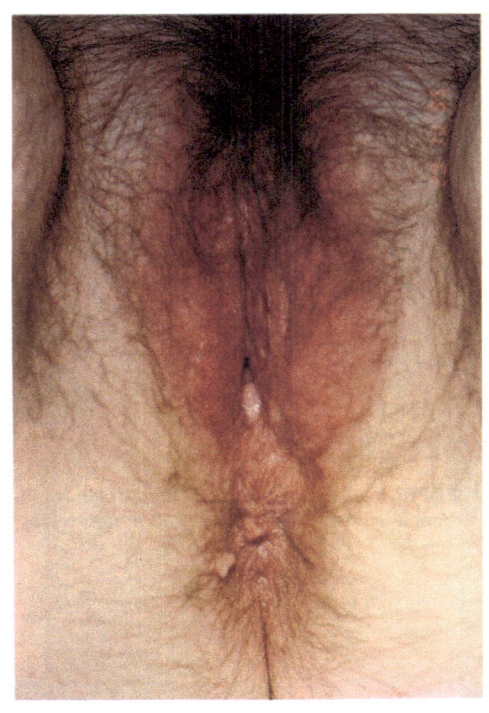

Fig. 160. Acute reddening with burning of the vulva for which no explanation was found. Contact allergy?

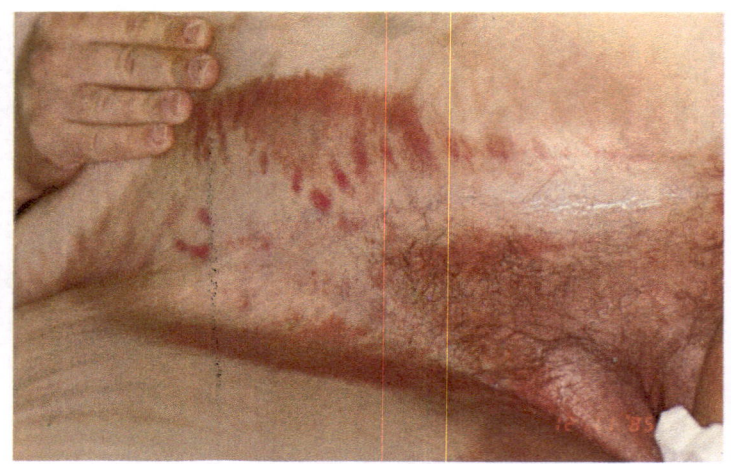

Fig. 161. Patient weighing 157 kg in labor; severe intertrigo in both groins. Fungal culture: *Rhodotorula rubra* (non-relevant)

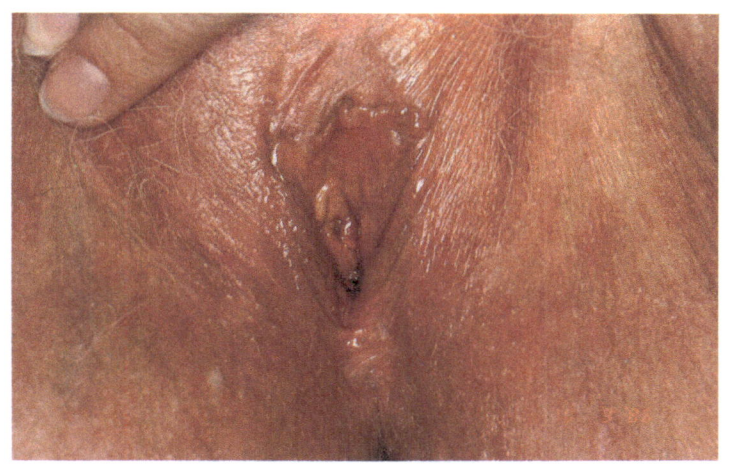

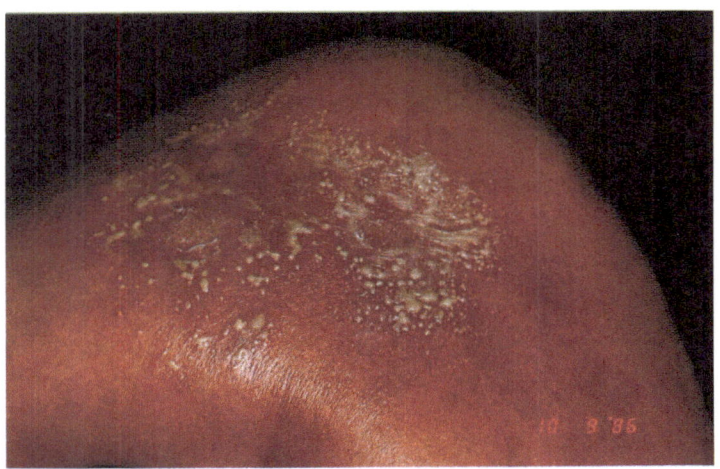

Fig. 162, 163. Pustular psoriasis (cf. Fig. 130–133 pp. 144 and 145)

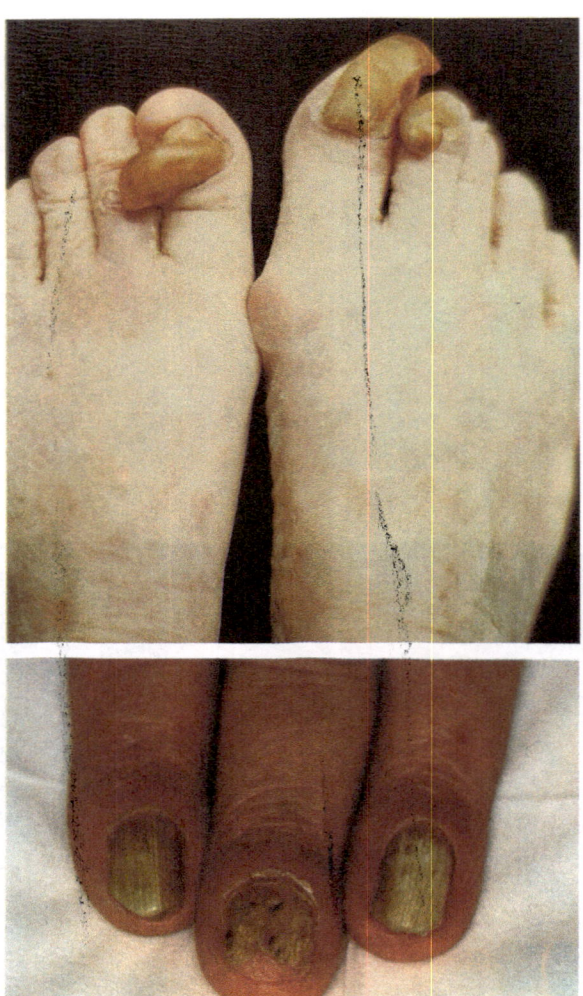

Fig. 164, 165. 80 year old woman's toe-nails, which had not been cut for 20 years, had withstood an attack of mycosis. However, mycosis of the nails for 20 years *(Candida tropicalis)* and recurrent vaginal mycosis *(Candida albicans)* in a 40 year old suggested impaired immunocompetence

11.8 Treatment

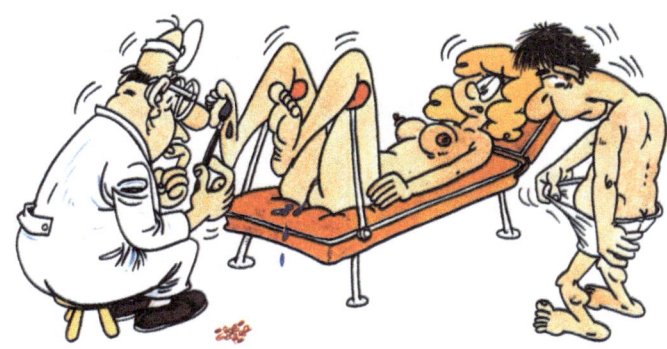

Fig. 166. Treatment with gentian violet is obsolete. (The picture was kindly made available to us by Dr. Ernst W. Loendersloot, Pieter Pauw Hospital, Wageninen, Netherlands.)

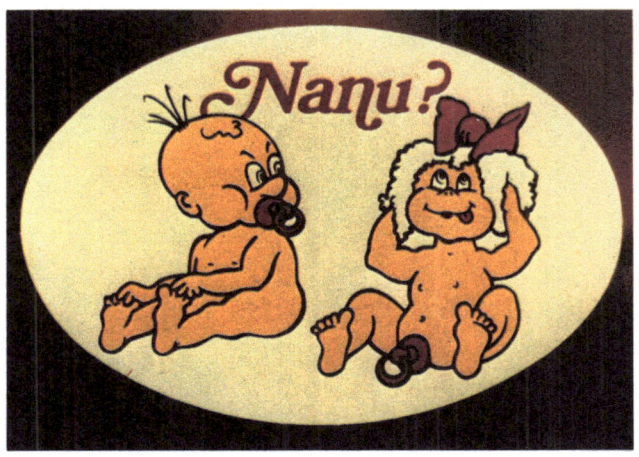

Fig. 167. Well, well! – Sources of reinfection which should be pointed out to patients with chronic recurrences

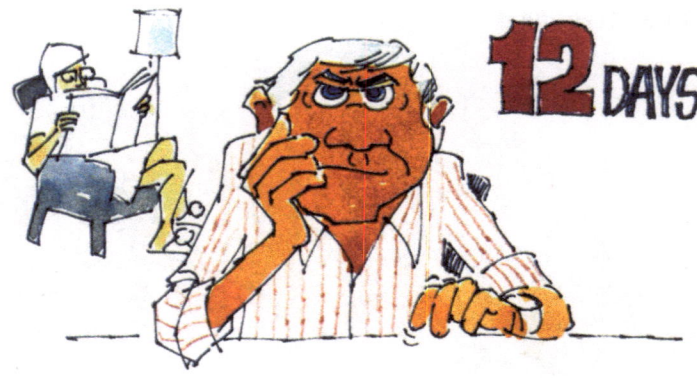

Fig. 168. Compliance ... (The picture was kindly made available to us by Dr. Ian Milsom, Department of Obstetrics and Gynecology, East Hospital, University of Göteborg, Sweden)

12 Subject Index

171